Bach Flower Remedies for Cats

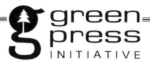

Bach Flower Remedies for Cats

Martin J. Scott and Gael Mariani

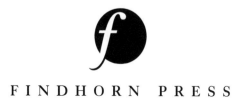

FINDHORN PRESS

First published by Findhorn Press 2007

ISBN: 978-1-84409-112-6

British Library Cataloguing-in-Publication Data.
A catalogue record for this book is available from the British Library.

Edited by Jane Engel
Cover design by Damian Keenan
Layout by Pam Bochel
Printed and bound in the USA

2 3 4 5 6 7 8 9 10 11 12 13 12 11 10

Published by
Findhorn Press
117–121 High Street,
Forres IV36 1AB
Scotland, UK

t +44(0)1309 690582
f +44(0)131 777 2711
e info@findhornpress.com
www.findhornpress.com

Contents

Acknowledgements   vii

Authors' Preface   ix

Foreword   xi

Chapter One: What are the Bach Flower Remedies?   1

Chapter Two: Cats and People   21

Chapter Three: The 38 Remedies   38

Chapter Four: Bach Flower Remedies in Specific Areas
of Feline Care   87

Chapter Five: The Last Goodbye: When We Lose a Cat   106

Chapter Six: Practicalities of giving Bach Remedies
to Cats   111

Chapter Seven: Frequently Asked Questions   118

Chapter Eight: Bach Flower Remedy Combinations   125

Chapter Nine: Looking After Your Cat's Physical Health
with Homeopathy   128

Chapter Ten: Case Histories from The S.A.F.E.R. Archives   135

Resources   150

Acknowledgements

The authors wish to express their sincere gratitude to all those who have helped with the long, difficult but always deeply satisfying process of researching the ways that Bach flower remedies and other flower essences can help animals. Special thanks must go to Richard Allport, MRCVS, Patron of the Society for Animal Flower Essence Research; Joanne Vyse-Killa VN; Julian Barnard; Jonathan Wright DVM and Melissa Wright; Colin Tennant and Ross McCarthy at the Canine and Feline Behaviour Association; and the many other friends and associates whose names would be too numerous to list here.

Finally, heartfelt thanks must go to the many cats and other animals who have proved our wisest and most valuable teachers over the years.

This book is dedicated to Chan, Rat and Pugsley.

Authors' Preface

The authors have been very involved for several years with Bach flower remedies and their uses in animal care. In 1998 we had the privilege of founding the first organisation in the world to specifically research and explore the ways that flower remedies could benefit animals: the Society for Animal Flower Essence Research (S.A.F.E.R.). Running the Society has been an exciting time and we are very indebted to the many valued associates and helpers who have joined us along the way. S.A.F.E.R. has been very fortunate in helping to promote the use of these profoundly effective and safe natural remedies for the benefit of many animals across the world. The tide is turning, and we are now beginning to see more and more use of flower remedies in animal rescue and rehabilitation centres to help the victims of cruelty, neglect and abandonment; in veterinary clinics to aid in the healing process for frightened, stressed or weak animals; in wild animal charity work, compassionate animal training centres, and last but not least in the homes of caring and dedicated pet owners everywhere who want to help their animals live a healthier, happier life. Bach flower remedies are truly one of the greatest gifts we have received from nature, and they are one of the greatest gifts we can give to any person we care for – whether that 'person' be a human loved one or a cherished animal friend and companion.

We have written this book for anyone interested in cats and their welfare, happiness and health. You may know nothing about the Bach remedies, may know a little or may have worked with the remedies for many years. Whatever your involvement with cats – veterinary science, feline behaviour counseling, rescue and rehabilitation, or the dedicated carer wishing to know more about how to improve the life of their feline companion – this book will give you a solid understanding of the many uses of Bach flower remedies in their care.

Foreword

By Richard Allport M.R.C.V.S

Vice-President of the British Association of
Homeopathic Veterinary Surgeons

B ach Flower remedies are safe and effective for humans and for animals of all species, but as a practising holistic vet I find cats are particularly responsive to the remedies. In this book you will find a well-researched and clear guide to the use of Bach Flower remedies for cats, as well as many fascinating insights into the world of cats in general. There has been a remarkable upsurge of interest in the field of natural therapies for pets in recent years, but a dearth of suitable books available to meet that interest.

This book is certainly going to be one that will help to fill that gap.

Chapter One

What are the
Bach Flower Remedies?

If you have picked up this book, you may already be familiar with this system of natural therapy pioneered by Dr Edward Bach (1886–1936). For those less familiar, the Bach flower remedies are a range of liquid remedies prepared from wild flowers. Their purpose is mainly in helping to heal negative emotional states: that is to say, states of mind and mood that cause suffering, or which are the result of suffering. These states of mind include emotions like sadness and despair, fear and anxiety, hostility and defensiveness, and the effects of emotional trauma past and present. The remedies come in liquid form, and are generally taken orally – although there are various other ways to use them, which we will be discussing in this book. They are 100% safe, inexpensive and widely available throughout the world. Animals respond to them particularly well, sometimes showing signs of improvement within minutes!

The Bach flower remedies are a strange paradox. They represent a fabulous technology of nature whose workings on living organisms are still something of a mystery to our crude human science. Yet for all its depth this natural healing resource is almost absurdly simple to use – so simple, in fact, that anyone can use the remedies without any previous study or knowledge. The results speak for themselves. For over seventy years now, this unassuming collection of gentle but powerful remedies has been quietly changing the lives of millions of people – and animals – across the world.

Many books have been written about the wide potential of Bach flower remedies to help with the problems we humans are so prone to. In this book we are going to shift the focus a little to look at how they can be used to help a fellow species we have brought into our human world: the cat, in all its many shapes and sizes. We'll examine the many ways that Bach remedies can change the lives of cats that are suffering from problems of the emotions, such as fear or stress or psychological tension stemming from past maltreatment.

Amongst plant-based natural remedies (herbs, essential oils, homeopathy etc.) Bach flower remedies occupy a special and unique place, not just because they are prepared like no other type of remedy but also because they are so simple to learn and use. It isn't possible to cause any problems with them, and any 'mistakes' you make by choosing an inappropriate remedy can easily and quickly be fixed simply by making a different choice and trying again. Flower remedies are a very forgiving subject to learn for the beginner. What this means is that even if you have never used them before, the information in this book will be more than enough to get you started using Bach flower remedies effectively to help the lives of cats or any other suffering creature, including humans. In a world where it seems so easy to do the wrong thing even with the best of intentions, Bach remedies seem to offer the impossible: here is something that can only do good. That's the beautiful reality of this system of therapy.

The life and legacy of Dr Edward Bach

Although it has its origins in history stretching back hundreds and possibly thousands of years, Dr Edward Bach is the person generally credited with the invention of the science of flower remedies. He was an English physician who gradually became increasingly disenchanted with conventional medical practice, and finally broke away, six years before his death, to develop a collection of special liquid-based remedies that were to become famous as the Bach Flower Remedies.

Edward Bach was an extremely caring and kind man who was deeply committed to relieving suffering in whatever way he could. His childhood love of nature, of plants and animals, was to be a guiding force throughout his medical career.

Early medical career

Bach qualified as a doctor in 1912. His health was never strong, and he was turned down for military service in World War 1 on medical grounds; it's unthinkable to contemplate that had it not been for this rejection, Bach might so easily have fallen with the millions of other victims of that conflict. We would never have inherited his legacy of the flower remedies! Bach spent the war years instead working at University College Hospital in his post of Assistant Bacteriologist. After the war he was appointed to the London Homeopathic Hospital. Homeopathic medicine was in those days, before the advent of antibiotics and the 'superdrug' era, a much more accepted and mainstream form of medicine than it is now. It was at the Homeopathic Hospital that Bach first encountered, and became captivated by, the teachings of homeopathy's founder, Dr Samuel Hahnemann. Bach's early writings, before the development of the Bach flower remedies, included The Relation of Vaccine Therapy to Homeopathy (1920), Intestinal Toxaemia in its Relation to Cancer (1924), The Problem of Chronic Disease (1927), and The Rediscovery of Psora (1928).

From early on in his medical work, Bach was aware of the important role of the psychological and emotional outlook of his patients. He observed that those patients with a generally positive and optimistic outlook on life, who were able to remain cheerful even in their sick state, tended to respond better to treatment and make a better recovery from illness. Meanwhile, those patients with a more pessimistic, gloomy, bitter or depressive outlook on life, perhaps despairing of ever getting well again, or being greatly affected by fear and anxiety about what was going to happen to them, tended to respond less well overall to treatment and were generally more prone to succumb to their illnesses. If they did recover, it was usually a much longer process.

Discovery of the mind-body connection

Dr Bach concluded from his observations that the emotions, psychological state, mindset and general attitude of a person must be a very significant factor in their overall state of wellbeing or constitutional strength. At the time his ideas were not taken seriously by the medical establishment, but in fact Bach had stumbled upon what is now an accepted concept in medicine, known by the rather long and unwieldy name of Psychoneuro-immunology (PNI for short). PNI is the study of how the state of mind can affect the state of physical health: for instance, the way a person suffering from chronic stress may have a lowered immune system and be prone to colds and viruses. Most doctors nowadays will readily accept the mind-body connection, as modern science has shown very conclusively that a poor state of mind will likely have an adverse effect on physical health sooner or later. Unhappy people become ill.

It's worth noting, however, that although the conventional medical scientific establishment now theoretically embraces this idea, in practice they have no real means of implementing it! Conventional therapies that act on the mind (mainly in the form of psychiatric drugs) can't have any significant PNI effect because they do not heal or cure psychological/emotional imbalances but instead simply bypass the symptoms by affecting brain chemistry. In general, once the drug treatment is stopped, the symptoms return within a short time showing that the root of the problem has not been touched. Almost a century after Dr Bach, our mainstream medical science is still cracking walnuts with sledgehammers and unable to grasp the simple, subtle beauty of something like flower remedies.

Creation of the bowel remedies

In his bacteriological work Bach discovered further evidence to link the physical and mental/emotional states of his patients: broadly classing people into groups according to temperament, he noticed that there were correlations between their psychological type and the state of their bowel flora, i.e. the bacterial state of their gut and faeces. Anxious types of people tended to show up one particular bowel 'picture'; angry types another, indecisive people another, and so on. On this basis, Bach created vaccinations derived from bowel flora and prescribed them largely according to patients' emotional states, with good results. However, Bach was dissatisfied. He was unhappy about working with the products of disease.

Discovery of homeopathy

Edward Bach's quest, from early on, was to find the most natural ways possible of relieving emotional suffering. When in 1919 he learned about homeopathy – at that time taken far more seriously by the conventional medical profession than it has been since the rise of the powerful pharmaceutical industry – he believed that he had discovered what he was looking for. He was attracted to homeopathy for its use of remedies that are nature-based, completely non-toxic and free of noxious chemical substances. He also approved of the fact that homeopathy's small innocuous remedies are mainly taken orally, as he disliked the idea of causing pain and injury to the patient by injecting them.

Bach attained fame as a homeopath when he created homeopathic versions from earlier bowel remedies: these were the Bowel Nosodes, derived from diseased human intestinal tissue and bowel flora but prepared homeopathically, extremely dilute and free from any noxious substances. The Bach Bowel Nosodes are still in use today as homeopathic remedies.

First plant remedies and discovery of the sunshine method

It was during his involvement with homeopathy that Dr Bach first experimented with making remedies from plants. These were homeopathic remedies, made by grinding (triturating) plant material and then subjecting it to the standard dilution/succussion homeopathic procedures to create different 'potencies' e.g. 30c, 200c, and so on. We know from his early writings, for instance, that his first version of the Impatiens remedy was 'triturated with sacc. lac. by hand... up to the seventh potency, after which succussion was adopted' (*Some New Remedies and New Uses*, published in *Homeopathic World,* February 1930).

Bach's homeopathic flower remedies were very effective at healing problems on both the physical and the mental/emotional levels: this early version of Impatiens, for example, was found effective in treating severe and acute pain as well as reducing accompanying fears and depression. Of course, this was nothing new to homeopathy, as a very large number of effective homeopathic remedies were already derived from flowers and plants.

Eventually, despite such successes, this highly idealistic doctor turned away from homeopathy altogether. He still wasn't satisfied, and wanted to find something that would come directly and unprocessed from nature, effective but completely gentle. And it wasn't long before he had found it. Sometime during 1930 he started using a very different and distinctly un-homeopathic system of making remedies. Instead of working in the laboratory as was – and still is – the practice in homeopathic pharmacy, Bach was now making his remedies out in the open air of the countryside.

His system was remarkably simple: he would place collected flower heads of a chosen type of flower into a glass bowl half-filled with ordinary water. The bowl containing water and flowers would be left to sit in the sun for two or more hours in a peaceful spot near where the flowers had been gathered. Then the water would be strained off, bottled and preserved with brandy. The flowers would be discarded. From these 'mother tincture' bottles, Bach would take two or three drops and place them in a second bottle, this time containing only neat brandy. From this bottle, containing the extremely dilute yet highly active flower-infused water, Bach would give a few drops at a time to patients suffering from emotional problems. Through extensive experimentation and trials he discovered that these new remedies were very effective and, just as importantly, completely safe.

The above method was known as the 'sunshine method'. Bach also employed a boiling method for making some of his remedies. With the boiling method, heat rather than sunlight was used to infuse the water with the qualities of the plant material. Afterwards, the water was strained off, the plant material thrown away, and from there the procedure was as the sunshine method of preparation.

Creation of the Bach flower remedies

In 1930 Bach closed his successful London medical practice, which had by then relocated to the prestigious site of Harley Street. He felt that he had reached the end of his involvement with conventional medicine as well as homeopathy. He now packed his bags and set off on what he believed to be the completion of his life's mission, exchanging a stable and lucrative career for a life of uncertainty and increasing poverty to seek out the 'healing herbs' that would gently address the emotions and mental states of his patients. He was convinced that in setting up a new system that would ease the mind, he could create a radical new approach to addressing physical illness too.

In the last six years of his life – for he died at the young age of fifty – Bach focused all his attention on the creation of this new system of therapy. He threw himself into his work, seldom resting. He spent a great deal of time walking around the wild parts of England and Wales, gathering material from flowers, shrubs and trees, and continually experimenting. By 1936, the year he died, Bach had created a collection of thirty-seven flower remedies, one remedy that did not come from the plant kingdom but which was uniquely prepared from a source of water with reputed healing properties (Rock Water), and one further remedy which was a special combination of five of the flowers. Nowadays this five-in-one combination goes by various names depending on which company produces it – Five-Flower Formula, Recovery Remedy, Rescue Remedy.

From the 12 healers to the 7 categories

Those who read Dr Bach's original writings will be able to trace the progress of his developing collection. He started slowly and carefully, examining different plants and developing his methodology as he went along. Between September 1928 and the summer of 1932 he selected twelve plants and created remedies from them. These were: Agrimony/Cerato/Centaury/Chicory/Clematis/Gentian/Impatiens/Mimulus/Rock Rose/Scleranthus/Vervain/Water Violet. Excited by his discoveries, he first wrote about these remedies in his 1933 publication *Twelve Healers,* which you can still read today. As he added more remedies to his list, he kept revising his system in more books and articles. To his *Twelve Healers* he added four 'helpers', then expanded those four to seven, and so on. Dr Bach probably had no idea that he would finally collect as many as 38. The last nineteen remedies in his collection, often referred to as 'the Second Nineteen' were developed in rapid succession in a huge burst of inspired activity between March and July 1935 – contrast this to the first nineteen, which had taken him more than six years to develop.

Not long before he died, Bach experimented with a way to categorise his remedies. Perhaps, because there were now so many of them, he was thinking that he needed a way to group them together to help people choose which one they needed. Based on his observations of people and their emotions and behaviour, he came up with 7 categories or headings:

1. **Fear**

2. **Uncertainty**

3. **Insufficient interest in present circumstances**

4. **Loneliness**

5. **Over-sensitivity to influences and ideas**

6. **Despondence and despair**

7. **Over-care for the welfare of others**

These categories are little used today. Many people find them confusing, and certainly, there are some problems with the system. For example, Dr Bach included his remedy Red Chestnut under **Fears**, when in fact it would have fitted much better under **Over-care for the welfare of others.** Red Chestnut helps when we are too worried about someone we love. Another example is the remedy Gorse, which can help with severe despair and feelings of hopelessness. Bach put this remedy under **Uncertainty** when it would have worked better under **Despondency and despair,** where (as we'll see later on) it would sit very well with remedies like Wild Rose. So while it's interesting to get a historical 'taste' of Dr Bach's original ideas, this experimental system of categories doesn't really work in practice. It works even less well for using Bach remedies with cats or other animals, whose psychology is a little different from our own.

In this book, we won't attempt to categorise or group the remedies in any particular way, but will simply examine each one in turn, in the order in which Dr Bach discovered them. Later in the book we'll take a detailed tour of all 38 Bach flower remedies, looking at the properties and uses of each one in turn and how they apply to helping cats. For the moment, below is a brief summary of the remedies as Dr Bach described them for helping human problems, giving a taste of what each one can be used for. If you have never read about the Bach remedies before, note how many of the painful states of mind, negative attitudes and out of balance behavioural tendencies listed below are extremely commonplace in everyday life; and think what kind of a world we could have without them!

Overview of the Bach flower remedies

(Presented in chronological order of their discovery by Dr Bach)

1. **Impatiens:** Forcing one's own fast pace onto others; impatient, intolerant of people's mistakes or slowness to understand.

2. **Mimulus: Everyday** fears of objects, people, circumstances; nervous anticipation of a coming event or situation.

3. **Clematis:** Daydreaming, disconnected from the present moment, ungrounded, 'not with it'.

4. **Agrimony:** Oversensitive to turmoil and quarrel; may seem outwardly cheerful but tormented by inner stress.

5. **Chicory:** Self-centred and attention-seeking relationship to others, tends to bind others to them.

6. **Vervain:** Overenthusiastic, (ideas or in general behaviour); hyper-energetic.

7. **Centaury:** Wants to please and serve, but too open to the demands of others; neglecting own needs.

8. **Cerato:** Inner uncertainty, lack of self-assurance, over-dependence on the advice of others.

9. **Scleranthus:** Vacillation between options, delay in making decisions; tendency to hesitate and be unsure of oneself.

10. **Water Violet:** Tendency to be too self-reliant to the point of shutting others out; closed off and hardened.

11. **Gentian:** Discouragement that may come with setbacks and difficulties; urge to give up or not try anything new.

12. **Rock Rose:** States of intense fear, terror and heightened nervousness.

13. **Gorse:** Hopelessness, despair, gloomy attitude and retreat from active engagement in the world.

14. **Oak:** States of stoic perseverance in the face of hardship and despair, leading to self-weakening and depletion of energy.

15. **Heather:** Tendency to be fixated on oneself, one's problems, etc.; not wanting to talk of anything else.

16. **Rock Water:** Tendency to be rigid, obsessive, stuck in a rut; too hard on oneself and trying to set an example.

17. **Vine:** Tendency to be a bully, domineering, bossy, taking control of people or situations.

18. **Olive:** Exhaustion and inability to attend to daily business.

19. **Wild Oat:** Lack of motivation and incentive plus uncertainty in choosing a 'life path'.

20. **Cherry Plum:** States of tension with fear of losing control of the rational mind: 'I'm going crazy'.

21. **Elm:** Feeling overwhelmed and overburdened by tremendous tasks, unable to meet the challenge any more.

22. **Aspen:** States of foreboding and vague haunting fears for which no explanation can be given.

23. **Chestnut Bud:** Difficulty absorbing new ideas or retaining lessons; tendency to repeat the same error.

24. **Larch:** Low self-esteem, lacking in confidence; sense that anything we try is doomed to failure.

25. **Hornbeam:** Mental fatigue, listlessness, procrastination in the face of duties.

26. **Willow:** Feeling not favoured by fate, or mistreated by others; developing bitterness and resentment

27. **Beech:** Tendency to be intolerant and critical of other people, with a judgmental outlook.

28. **Crab Apple:** Unable to rise above 'shameful' aspects of the self and despairing over them.

29. **Walnut:** Oversensitive and vulnerable to outside impressions, too affected by things.

30. **Holly:** Easily upset and irritated by vexing and annoying circumstances; angry outlook.

31. ***Star of Bethlehem:*** Burdens of grief, trauma and shock and their after-effects.

32. ***White Chestnut:*** Mental agitation, pre-occupation or intense worries that seem to take over the whole mind and are hard to 'switch off.'

33. ***Red Chestnut:*** Too bound up in worrying over the wellbeing of someone close; frustrated sense of helplessness.

34. ***Pine:*** States of guilt and self-reproach, tendency to feel responsible or take on board blame for every little thing.

35. ***Honeysuckle:*** Living in the past, belief that happiness can never be repeated again in the future.

36. ***Wild Rose:*** Apathy and withdrawal, sense of giving up, wanting to retreat and fade away.

37. ***Mustard:*** Withdrawal into depression and gloominess, lack of joy in life.

38. ***Sweet Chestnut:*** Unbearable anguish and despair, deep emotional pain, sense of futility and joylessness.

Between them, the Bach flower remedies cover an enormous range. Because they can be combined together, there are a virtually infinite number of possible ways they can work together to address the problems of any individual sufferer. This makes them an extremely individualised and personalised therapy, whether used to help a human or any other animal.

Tragically, Dr Bach was a very sick man in those last years while the flower remedies were being created. The cancer that had nearly killed him during his twenties had finally caught up with him again. It may be that Bach had burned himself out working so hard; or perhaps the reason he had worked so furiously to complete his system was that he knew he had limited time. We shall never know. When he died in November 1936 he was virtually penniless, having invested everything he had into his project. His only source of hope was his faith that his system of healing with flower remedies would bring relief to a suffering world.

It actually took many years for the Bach flower remedies to become widely known and used across the world. Bach's immediate followers, including Nora Weeks and Victor Bullen, kept on the Oxfordshire country house that had been Bach's base at the end of his life, and set up what is now the Edward Bach Foundation/Bach Centre. The production and promotion of the Bach flower remedies gradually grew up into a successful business, reaching a high level of popularity from the 1970s and 80s onwards when there was a surge in public interest in complementary therapies. The original business was sold to the homeopathic pharmaceutical company, Nelsons, for a large sum of money and a new division, Nelson Bach, was formed that has transformed the Bach flower business into a huge global industry. Meanwhile, other companies started producing their own versions of the Bach remedies. One such company is Ainsworths, another homeopathic pharmacy. Another Bach flower remedies producer is Healing Herbs Ltd, which has deliberately eschewed the mass-production path taken by the larger companies and adheres to the pure methods of Dr Bach, producing everything by hand and using only the purest, finest, organic ingredients. Many people believe that the final result of such an approach is a superior, more effective remedy.

Dr Bach's view of health and illness

Bach not only saw his remedies as important for helping with emotional problems, he also regarded them as very important in the context of medical treatment and physical health. This idea was based on his observations of sick patients: the happier and more cheerful patients tended to do better, while the unhappy or pessimistic, angry, despairing patients tended to be more vulnerable to their illness. In his Wallingford lecture, given on his 50th birthday shortly before he died, Bach outlined the four ways of using the remedies:

1. **Prevention of ill health**
   Keeping strong in mind/emotions by treating mental/ emotional states as they arise. This can have a very powerful effect on our general immunity to illnesses, and our constitutional strength. Bach was one of the first doctors to gain such an accurate insight into the medical importance of a positive mental attitude.

2. **Help stop illness at onset**
   Dr Bach believed that by keeping the emotions bright and healthy, threatened illnesses could be prevented from developing; or at least, their effect could be reduced.

3. **Help during illness, once it has begun**
   Dr Bach had seen the importance of helping sick patients regain and maintain their optimism and cheerfulness. He had noticed that happier people would recover much better from illness and respond better to treatment. It follows that using the Bach flower remedies can help the sick to recover more quickly, not by treating the direct cause of the illness but by supporting the patient's mental strength, optimism and resolve.

4. **Help with character traits that bring unhappiness**
   Dispositions of character that cause problems for the sufferer can be gently transformed, allowing a happier and freer personality to emerge.

The Bach flower remedies: what they are, how they work

For many people, it's not important to understand how Bach remedies work, or even whether they've been 'proven' to work by scientists. Many of us are simply content to use them and see the benefits they offer to us, our loved ones and our companion animals. Indeed, there is a large and fast-growing body of anecdotal evidence to support the beliefs of millions of people that Bach flower remedies really do work as claimed. They are used across the world by many vets, doctors and other healthcare professionals who would have little interest in them if they weren't getting results! In Cuba, for instance, Bach remedies are now integrated into the national health system.

Nonetheless, like alternative and complementary therapy in general, Bach remedies are still an area of controversy. For all their millions of satisfied users, among the conventional medical establishment there is still much resistance to the idea that these odd little bottles can really contain anything worthwhile. Many readers of this book, who may never have seen a Bach remedy in action, may be hungry for more information that could persuade them to take this therapy seriously. So it would seem like a wasted opportunity merely to use this book to 'preach to the converted' and not to try to take a slightly deeper look for the benefit of readers who may be new to all this.

To the question 'do they work?' the answer is an emphatic yes, they do. The efficacy of Bach flower remedies is now well established through decades of reliable anecdotal evidence as well as a growing number of scientific studies (mainly on people). As to how they work, we'll come right out and say that nobody has ever demonstrated scientifically how, exactly, Bach remedies are able to have the effect they do. However, there is enough peripheral scientific knowledge to be able to piece together a pretty good layperson's picture of what's going on inside the body when we take a Bach remedy or give one to a cat.

The tired old placebo argument

One of the arguments often 'trundled out' against Bach remedies is the claim that their apparent benefits are really nothing more than a placebo effect. This is a recognised effect whereby a person suffering from a given problem can be made better by giving them a 'placebo' remedy. A placebo remedy doesn't contain anything that might help – it might just be a little unmedicated sugar pill, or even just a glass of plain water – but works on the basis of the patient's trust and faith in their doctor and their belief that they will get better. And indeed, it's sometimes possible to 'trick' people into getting better this way. When drugs are being tested in medical trials, placebos are used as controls to show by comparison that the drug really works. Humans receiving placebo remedies usually show a 10% improvement on these 'blanks'. This is a fascinating insight into the power of the mind.

But is this the way Bach remedies work? The easiest way to argue against this theory is when we point out that Bach remedies help animals. You can't 'trick' an animal into getting better. In veterinary medical trials where drugs are being tested on animals, control groups are used to compare the progress of the animals given the drugs to those that are given nothing, but none of the animals given these 'blank' remedies show any placebo effect. With Bach remedies, the fact that a cat, dog, horse or bird can be helped is strong evidence that the Bach remedies really do work.

Bach remedies compared to other types of plant remedy

To get an understanding of how the Bach remedies work and what they really are, it's a good idea first of all to distinguish them clearly from other types of natural remedy that may at first sight seem very similar. Bach flower remedies are often confused with some of their cousins, other types of remedies derived from the plant kingdom, As we'll see, they're really very different indeed!

It's very easy to think of the Bach flower remedies as a type of herbal medicine. Another misconception is the confusion between flower remedies and essential oils.

Both herbal remedies and aromatherapy oils use the active biochemical properties of plants to bring about chemical changes to the body (affecting physical symptoms) and brain (affecting mental/emotional symptoms). Herbal remedies take the chemical properties of plants straight from nature, while essential oils are distilled and highly concentrated, and must generally be used very diluted. While these types of remedies aren't as powerful or as toxic as modern medical drugs, some care needs to be exercised in using them. Essential oils, for instance, must usually be heavily diluted before use, and users are advised to carry out 'patch tests' on small areas of skin before treatment, in case of irritation. It's also unsafe to give essential oils orally to any animal. Another problem with herbal remedies, recently the subject of media discussion, is that some of them can interact adversely and unpredictably with certain medical drugs.

However, although they also come from plants, Bach flower remedies differ very greatly from either of these types of remedy. They are 100% safe, they do not contain material doses of plant chemicals, and they can be used alongside any form of medication without any risk of adverse interactions. Completely unlike their herbal cousins, Bach flower remedies contain nothing of the chemical properties of the source plant. Spectroscopic analysis shows that Bach flower remedies are physically dilute to the point that they contain literally 'nothing' that can (using existing technologies) be measured or quantified, i.e. not one molecule of the source substance. This is why they have none of the perfume of an essential oil. They contain ONLY the water and the preservative that keeps the water in good condition (usually brandy). This means they are absolutely safe and non-toxic. It also could be taken to mean that they are absolutely useless! But practice shows them to be highly effective. How, then, do we explain how Bach remedies work?

Understanding energy

Bach flower remedies are what we call a dynamic therapy, as opposed to a material therapy that uses something tangible and measurable, e.g. chemicals, to operate. The Bach flowers use a particular form of subtle energy to work on our bodies and minds.

Living beings – including ourselves and our cats – are very much energetic in nature. What does this mean? No, it doesn't mean we're always jumping around and full of beans; it means that these fleshy bodies we inhabit are actually made of nothing more or less than energy. Every molecule of a living organism vibrates at a particular energetic (electromagnetic) frequency, and every living being has an unseen yet very real energy or bio-electrical field, which surrounds, penetrates and permeates the physical body. In fact, this energy field *is* the physical body!

Sounds bizarre? Well, it sounded bizarre to physicists too, before Albert Einstein's physics revolution in 1905. Nowadays it's bread-and-butter knowledge that energy fields are actually more fundamental to reality than our normal concept of 'matter', and that visible matter is no more than a state of energy in varying stages of density. Physics shows, for example, that the chair you are sitting on to read this book is itself nothing more than a very dense conglomeration of energetic subatomic particles and that the interaction between it and your body – the fact that it supports you and you don't fall through it – is actually down to the interaction of the chair's and your body's respective electro-magnetic fields.

For a practical understanding of this idea, try pressing two magnets together. You'll find they either attract or repel each other, depending on which poles you bring together. This repulsion is basically what keeps you from falling through the earth! Due to these same forces, when you turn this page, your fingers will not be physically touching the paper but rather it will be the energy field of your fingertips interacting with the energy field of the paper that enables you to move them. In other words, energy underlies and dictates all physical relationships between things, and is utterly crucial to the existence and stability of matter. What we sense with our five physical senses and feel with our emotional capacity is only the reflection, the by-product, of an unseen, supersensible realm of energy.

With the advance of scientific understanding in the modern age comes the growing realisation among scientists that the truth about nature, the planet and the wider cosmos is much 'weirder' than we ever thought. One of the latest developments at this time has been the increasing acceptance among cosmologists that most of the matter in the universe is composed of so-called 'dark matter'. The staggering thing about dark matter is that is seems to contain no chemical elements at all – no molecules of anything! Yet this radical suggestion is gaining ground. If it's true, it not only overturns many of the traditionally held 'truths' about physics and chemistry, it also makes something like a flower remedy seem far less weird, and far more conventionally acceptable, by comparison!

Scepticism and science

Modern biology is forced to follow where modern physics leads, and to a large extent it does. Unfortunately, one major corner of the biology world, the medical establishment, remains dominated by thinking that is now very outdated (by at least a century). It's this backward-looking conventional thinking that puts up the big barriers to any form of energy therapy or medicine. It states that there must be molecules of a substance for that substance to 'be something' and have an effect. If there's 'nothing' in a remedy, according to this understanding it can't work and any reported effects must be due to the placebo effect, i.e. a kind of faith healing.

But we already know that the placebo effect can't account for the beneficial effects of Bach remedies on animals. Furthermore, where does this leave common medical technologies such as X-rays, ultrasound or lasers? There's 'nothing' in them either, yet they are well established at the heart of medical practice. Clearly, something else is going on.

Digital biology

Cutting-edge 'digital biology' sheds light on unanswered questions in science by revealing the nature of electromagnetic molecular signalling: that is, the way that information passes through the physical body. After eight years of research and in the course of thousands of replicated experiments, the late French scientist Dr Jacques Benveniste and his team at DigiBio Laboratories were able to transfer specific molecular energy signals onto a computer sound card. By playing these signals as sound (energy) waves to samples of material, they were able to lead receptor cells to 'believe' and act as though they were in the presence of the original molecules from which the signals had been gathered, even though they were not physically present.

In other words, one could say that biological systems function rather like radio sets, by a process of co-resonance. If you have a radio receiver tuned to a certain frequency, say BBC Radio 2, you will receive that signal from the transmitter vibrating at the same frequency. You won't find any molecules of Radio 2 in the miles of air between your radio and the broadcasting station! The wave that carries the information is a form of energy.

These are likely to be the kinds of activities going on in the body when we take a flower remedy, the sending of bio-resonant energy waves through tissue and water carrying digital healing information. According to this model, the Bach flower remedies operate by bio-electrical resonance.

Think of it as a subtle, hi-tech version of herbalism that dispenses with the crudeness of molecular chemistry. One could liken the difference to that between a mechanical instrument (akin to herbalism) and an electronic one (akin to Bach flower remedies). If herbs and essential oils are an abacus, Bach flower remedies are a high-performance computer.

Uploads and downloads

Bach flower remedies make use of the ability of simple water to retain or 'upload' the energy frequencies of a flower. When we take a Bach remedy, or give some to a cat, we are in a sense 'downloading' that information back into their system. The body's own energy system conducts the information in the form of very subtle energy waves which travel through water and tissue. The energy field of the flower, carried in the water, is able to interact with the field of the recipient and influence its state. This effect then filters down, by a complex process of electrochemical conversions, into the conscious mind as improved mental/emotional/psychological wellbeing.

Each different type of flower has a slightly different energy and carries slightly different 'information' into our system. This means that each of the 38 Bach remedies is able to address and influence a slightly different aspect of our energy field. But what they all have in common is that they are capable of healing blockages and imbalances at the highest and most subtle level of our being and that of animals. This highest level is the realm of the mind and emotions, the psychological state – or, if we dare to risk using such terms, the 'heart and soul'.

Bach remedies in the future

In distant years to come, we may find flower remedy therapy entering a complete new phase of scientific development. It may even one day be possible to convert the energy forms of Bach flower remedies into sound waves, permitting us to play them through speakers, or even construct 'scanners' that patients could simply walk through to receive the healing benefits. Once converted to a digital medium that our computers could read, we could download flower remedies from the Internet, carry them around on recording media such as CDs, and email them to each other! At present, the state of the art remains the highly effective and perfectly practical liquid format originally devised by Dr Edward Bach.

Bach remedies and animals

Helping animals, including cats, has always been a potential part of the scope of Bach flower therapy. From the early days, Dr Bach saw that his remedies would benefit not just humans but all living creatures, even ailing plants. However, it is only relatively recently that practitioners of Bach therapy have begun to turn their attentions to the remedies' uses in helping animals. Attitudes to animals have changed enormously over the last few decades, with a substantial increase in the recognition of, and respect for, their psychological and emotional complexity. One of the species of animal that can most benefit from this healthy modern trend is the cat. The rest of this book is devoted to exploring the many ways that Bach flower remedies can be used to enhance the lives of our feline friends.

Chapter Two

Cats and People

The magical, mysterious history of the cat

The cat is an animal that has long been associated with mystery and magic – and not always to its benefit. This far-reaching historical association has its roots in ancient Egypt, widely believed to be the birthplace of the cat, as we know it today. The ancient Egyptians venerated the cat as a symbol both of fertility and the moon, two natural phenomena that they realised were strongly interrelated in a number of ways. The Egyptians worshipped the cat in the form of the goddess Bastet, who originated in the delta of the Nile. Originally, Bastet took the form of a lioness; later on, after the domestication of the cat around 3,500 years ago when cats, frequenting the cities that were sprouting up all across Egypt, began to integrate more into human society, Bastet took on the aspect of cat, as we know it. Bastet had her own temple, and a whole city, Bubastis, was built in her honour and that of the cat. On a special day each year, some 700,000 people – much of the population of Egypt at that time – would come by the boatload to worship Bastet at her temple beside the Nile.

As time went by, the cat came to enjoy similar sacred status in many other ancient cultures, such as in Palestine. In Buddhist cultures it was venerated as a guardian of the temples and of the souls of the dead. To this day, you will usually find cats around if you visit one of the Buddhist temples of south-east Asia, where many people still uphold the traditional belief that the souls of good men are transmuted into feline form.

By the time the cat had begun to appear in ancient Greek and Roman cultures, it came not simply as an animal but with a whole baggage of religious mythology that fitted in quite neatly alongside the deities of the time – Diana, the huntress and moon goddess of the Romans, and Artemis, who served a similar role as the fertility goddess of the ancient Greeks. In other respects, the cat was increasingly seen by these fast-growing cultures as a very practical and useful animal, primarily due to its important role in pest control.

With the spread of the Roman Empire into Europe, which was to develop into the spread of Christendom, came the rise of the cat in Britain, France and elsewhere. When the cat 'invaded' Europe on the Roman ships, it brought with it the sacred heritage that had been formed back in Egypt. Pre-Christian Europe had long been steeped in fertility magic and ritual, and the cat soon came to be regarded with the same kind of symbolic significance that the Egyptians had attributed to it. Cats featured heavily in the magic and ritual of fertility worship across Europe – sometimes in a macabre form such as in the corn ceremonies of old southern France when cats were ritually put to death as a sacrifice to the gods overseeing the success of the wheat crops.

As the centuries rolled by, the positive aspects of cat mythology turned sour in Western Europe. With the rise of patriarchal Christianity and the Catholic Inquisition came the ruthless dismantling of old pagan beliefs and religious structures. The tradition of the divine feminine was stamped out and the idea of fertility goddess worship was vilified. This was the start of a dark period in the cat's history that was to last for a long time, for by medieval times the cat was being regarded in a whole new light: not only as a tool of the Devil, but as the Devil incarnate.

Cat hatred was soon to reach a terrifying peak, and with it the hatred and persecution of anything related to the 'old ways' of pagan culture and nature-worship – particularly if carried out by women. Heretic trials often featured cats, and any woman seen showing kindness to a cat could be branded a witch and cruelly executed. Even just enjoying the companionship of a cat was considered a mark of Satan. In England at the height of the witchcraft persecution, around the late 16th century, a woman could be burned simply for placing wool in a cat's basket to make a comfortable bed for the animal. Cats themselves became the focus of ritual execution, and it became customary for the hapless animals to be burned alive at religious festivals, fetes and country fairs. These traditions carried on for many years and led to the massacre of hundreds of thousands of cats.

One of the most notorious events to take place during those cat-hating centuries in Europe was the decree issued by the Lord Mayor of London in 1348 that all cats should be exterminated completely in order to purge the land of evil. Apart from the cruelty and barbarism involved, this may also have been one of the most unwise public health policies ever implemented. The resulting cull of thousands upon thousands of cats only led to a large increase in the rat population. When trading ships from the east brought with them the bubonic plague, the disease began to spread at an alarming rate. It was the rats that helped to spread 'the black death' so far and wide, and before long the plague had wiped out nearly half the human population of Europe. This must surely be one of the great examples of how human foolishness has always tended not only to affect the animal world but ultimately to rebound back on us!

It was only several centuries later that mankind finally realised the important role of the cat in combating the disease (especially following the discovery of bacteria by Louis Pasteur in the 1800s), and cats began to lose their witchcraft stigma, were recognised as a very clean and useful animal and were again allowed to share the lives of humans. The relationship between the two species has been quite stable since that time. The first major cat show in the UK was held in London's Crystal Palace in 1871, and this event marks the beginning of the rebirth of popular acceptance of the cat in Britain.

A shared history: the ancient origins of flower remedies

Interestingly, the often-troubled history of the cat has a great deal in common with the fascinating and little-known historical origins of the flower remedy. While Dr Edward Bach is credited with having created the flower remedy as we know it today, in fact there is a good deal of evidence to show that remedies using the subtle energies of plants and flowers stretches right back through history, all the way to the old alchemists of ancient Egypt and Arabia. Dr Bach, with his keen interest in Freemasonry and ancient cultures, may in fact have been consciously drawing on a whole tradition of natural healing that began in Egypt and spread to ancient China, then was later imported into Europe as an indirect result of the medieval crusades.

In just the same way as cats became stigmatised as satanic, the traditions of herbal folklore and alchemy came to be regarded with serious suspicion and their practitioners branded as heretics. Many early European scientists, pioneers of modern physics in that they sought to understand the energetic, sub-atomic root of all matter – how and why things really worked and what they were made of at the deepest levels – lived in constant terror of being caught by the Inquisition and burned at the stake. One such unfortunate scientist was the Italian mathematician Giordano Bruno, burned at the stake in the year 1600 for dabbling in scientific practices frowned upon by the Church.

Centuries later, Dr Edward Bach may have been secretly concerned about the dark and mysterious heritage from which he developed his flower remedies. Could this have been the reason why, shortly before his death in 1936, he deliberately burned all his research notes? This event, tragic for those of us nowadays who wish to understand exactly how he came upon his amazing ideas, is as deeply shrouded in mystery as the fascinating shared history of the cat and the flower remedy.

In a very real sense, when we bring cats and flower remedies together in our modern world, we are reuniting two ancient, sacred and mysterious relics of a fascinating though often dark past. Both the cat and the flower remedy have been the object of persecution in their time; both have witnessed the cruel torture of the innocent by ruthless forces intent on domination. To bring them both together now in this more enlightened age is a celebration of the good in ancient cultures, as well as a tribute to two survivors who made it through the dark times!

Cats today

In the modern age, cats are one of the most popular pets. It has been estimated that the cat population has increased by 40% in recent years in the UK and continues to swell by around 2% a year. The same kinds of increases are being seen in other countries, such as the USA. This rate is over double the rate of increase in dog ownership.

One of the reasons for the cat's great popularity is its flexibility and adaptability. It has proved able to live in a wide variety of conditions and environments. Most cat owners are able to accommodate their cat's needs quite well, treating it as a loved member of their family while also allowing it freedom to roam as it pleases and to express his predatory nature. This dual quality is a hallmark of the cat: on the one hand it is generally sociable with humans and provides warmth and companionship for many people; yet on the other hand they are fiercely independent and have lost little of their wildness (in fact they cannot truly be said to have been 'domesticated'). Understanding this wild streak in the cat is very necessary to knowing what cats are about. The cat has been subjected to far less artificial genetic mutation (otherwise known as breeding) at the hands of humans than the dog: it has had relatively little breeding for type and virtually none for task (we have not created specific breeds of 'working cats', as in dogs and horses). The cat's physical and behavioural characteristics are almost unaltered compared to those of its wild ancestors and cousins. Even in the domestic situation, the cat continues to be what has been called 'arguably the most successful mammalian predator the world has ever seen.'

The independent cat

Probably the one trait that most sets the cat apart from the dog and the horse, the two other animals that mankind has most widely introduced into our culture, is its powerful and resilient spirit of independence. This aspect of the cat no doubt accounts also for why we tend to be either 'cat lovers' or 'cat haters' – while many people have a deep admiration for the animal's independence, others are repelled by it. This possibly says more about them than about the cat, and it is interesting to note that some of the world's most famous dictators, men like Alexander the Great, Napoleon Buonaparte and Adolf Hitler, all professed a strong dislike of cats. Hitler was, incidentally, very fond of dogs, and one could speculate at length on the real reasons why some people prefer one species to the other!

Cats and dogs

Many people find that in a moment of upheaval, such as a divorce or an unsettled phase in the household, where the home loses its atmosphere of stability, their cats may simply leave and set up home elsewhere. Sometimes they may return when things are better, or else they may stay away for good. In some cases they may settle only a short distance from their previous home, perhaps in the same street. The previous owners may see the cat around, but he shows no inclination to return 'home'. This kind of behaviour differs significantly from that of dogs. The family dog will tend to stick with the pack through thick and thin, often absorbing stresses and perhaps even becoming miserable and neurotic, but not running away unless situations become very extreme (even then, most stray dogs have not run away, but have been deliberately abandoned). The contrast between the 'faithful dog' and the 'independent cat' has led to the popular idea that cats are quite mercenary and self-seeking by nature. This is placing a value judgment on the cat that is completely unwarranted: in fact their behaviour simply reflects what they are, a solitary, relatively non-social, very self-sufficient and independent predator.

One of the possible reasons for the increase in the popularity of cats as pets is linked to the fact that families are tending more towards being double-income families with more married women breaking away from the traditional housewife role. When the couple is out at work and the children at school, the home is empty for much of the day. Many people feel they cannot take on the responsibility of a dog, which will need to be taken out for walks in order to have its exercise and relieve itself. As a result, many people who would really rather have a dog end up getting a cat as a compromise, literally as a dog substitute. This pet substitution is in theory no bad thing, given the fact that the cat is more independent than the dog and can be much more of a 'low-maintenance' pet, like a goldfish or a mouse. However, this substitution can also lead to problems when people fail to take into account just how unlike cats are from dogs. One animal behaviourist of the authors' acquaintance is now seeing many more cats than dogs in her practice, and the most common lesson that her human clients need to be taught is that 'a cat is not a dog'. This echoes the words of T.S. Eliot in his poem *The Ad-dressing of Cats:*

Again I must remind you that a dog's a dog, a cat's a cat!

The social cat

Despite its relatively non-social nature compared to dogs and horses, the cat should not necessarily be perceived as a complete loner. Cats in the domestic environment can form strong social bonds with one another and with other animals, notably dogs. These kinds of social bonds are not restricted to the domestic environment. Groups of feral cats (cats once domesticated, but which have reverted back to a near-wild state) will often form colonies and live together. This tends to happen when resources are abundant, and there is less pressure on each individual cat to mind their personal survival. These groups are often largely female, with queens sharing mothering duties and tending to each other's kittens. This feline social group, or matriarchal colony, is reminiscent of the lion prides of Africa, one of the very few examples of highly social cats in the wild. It's important to note that in such colonies of cats, it is the group that decides whether a new cat is to be accepted or rejected. This way there are far fewer disputes amongst feral cats than in artificial domestic situations where it is humans who clumsily attempt to bring cats together and force them to co-exist.

The indoor cat

Many professional cat behaviourists report that they see a disproportionate number of cats kept permanently indoors compared with free-range pets. As one might expect from an animal like the cat, behaviour problems often result from being kept isolated from their natural outdoor lifestyle.

Reasons for keeping a cat confined indoors may vary. In some cases it may be out of concern for the cat's safety, if perhaps home is a very busy urban area with a lot of traffic posing a risk to free-ranging cats, or a high-rise apartment where the cat would not be physically able to come and go. In other cases it may be due to the owner's perception of the cat: some owners of indoor cats are less willing to embrace the idea of their pet as an independent animal that needs to remain in charge of its lifestyle and must have freedom to express natural behaviours.

Cats can become bored, unfulfilled and stressed due to their confinement and inability to express their natural ways. Deprived of the natural occupation of hunting and territory surveillance, the indoor cat may express his predatory side by playing ambush/attack games with humans in the household. This can occasionally cause problems, especially when the cat plays too roughly and people are scratched or bitten. Damaged furniture is a common problem, as cats seek to distract themselves by scratching things. Stressed cats may also start scent-marking the inside of the house, especially entire males. This is likely to be accentuated by the nearby presence of other cats occupying the territory. The lack of proper mental stimulation for the indoor cat, combined with the stress of being kept in can, in some extreme cases, lead to stress-related fur pulling, over-grooming and self-mutilation.

Solving problems due to confinement will always involve some kind of management of the cat's lifestyle. Owners who keep their cats confined indoors may have to start letting them out more, perhaps fitting a cat flap to allow the cat to come and go more independently (although this can also create new problems, with neighbouring cats coming in and invading the territory). Owners living in high-rise apartments or very busy city environments, where the cat cannot come and go, should consider interacting with their cats more, playing with them and giving them toys to stimulate them: mouse toys, ping-pong balls, crumpled newspaper, crinkly pieces of silver foil, hanging ropes, hide-and-seek games, find-the-food games, are all ways that the cat can amuse itself and interact positively with the owner. A scratching-post is also an important accessory for cats confined indoors, and can help to save the furniture and curtains! Some companies produce cat scratching-posts impregnated with the scent of the herb cat-nip, which is attractive to cats. This may be useful if your cat doesn't otherwise show any interest in scratching-posts – however it may need to be replaced periodically, as the scent can fade with time.

Lack of sunlight is a potential hazard to the health of any animal kept indoors. Indoor cats may become listless, run down and generally less healthy due to being deprived of natural sunlight. Owners should try to find a way to expose indoor cats to sunlight whenever possible. A sunny windowsill can provide a cat with a healthy place to rest and absorb the sun's goodness (while also being able to look out at the activities of the world). However, cats should also be given the choice to retreat to a shady area if they desire.

Understanding your cat: Feline body language and communication

Like many animals, cats use many body signals to communicate with one another, and in order to understand how our cats are feeling, and what they're thinking, it's quite important to be able to read and interpret this visual form of language.

A cat that feels threatened

When cats are feeling threatened and acting in a defensively aggressive manner, they will do what they can to make themselves seem bigger and more imposing. They arch their backs, bristle their fur and can look twice their normal size. If the threat continues, the next stage in the cat's defensive strategy is to display teeth and claws; the ultimate stage is to use them, and cats will not hesitate to do so if pushed. For this reason, humans should be aware of the signals of a defensive-aggressive cat, and should not corner or intimidate them.

Threatened but submissive

A cat that is very threatened but adopts submissive behaviour is deferring to the threatening party, showing that they're backing down and not interested in a fight. Such cats will tend to make themselves as small as possible; if the threat is maintained, their main interest is escape, if possible. A submissive cat has a much higher threshold of aggression than a more confident cat – that is to say, it takes a lot more to make the nervous cat turn and fight. Only when all escape is cut off, and the threatening party still does not back down, will the cat resort to defensive aggression. Some cats in this position will roll over on their backs; however this is not to be interpreted as the absolute submissiveness of a dog that rolls on his back – the cat is still liable to strike, grasping any approaching hand with all four paws and delivering a strong bite.

When humans get it wrong!

When approaching an unfamiliar cat, especially one that may be nervous, it's important not to press yourself on it or stare it in the eyes! Most species automatically recognise a steady, unblinking stare as something only a dominant and confident animal will do. Humans, who are as a species very out of touch with their own body signals, not to mention those of other species, tend to overlook this fact! Many people try to impose themselves on cats, and such pushy behaviour will frequently drive cats away. Interestingly, the cat will often tend to be attracted to the person in the household who least tries to push themselves on him.

Reading the cat's eyes

Many people believe that cat behaviour can be read in the eyes. However, going by eyes alone can be misleading. Narrowing or widening of the eyes can variously mean the cat is angry, fearful or just curious! Pupils will dilate if cat is frightened or feeling aggressive. However, they can also become dilated due to the joy of seeing a friend, or owner. Pupil dilation also depends on the amount of light present: pupils tend to be larger in the dark, contracted in the light. Thus, there are no hard and fast rules. What a cat is communicating with his eyes needs to be read in the context of the situation and the rest of his body language.

Ear signals

Ear signals are often a better clue to the cat's frame of mind or behaviour mode, especially when read in the context of other signals. Ears perked up straight and alert, with pupils dilated to let in the maximum of light and enhance vision, will be seen in cats that are hunting or playing. A cat that is annoyed will tend to turn his ears back, often with a constriction of the pupils and the whiskers bristling forward. Combined with bristling fur, arched back (both designed to make the cat look as big as possible) and bared teeth, the signs of a defensively aggressive cat are quite unmistakable. Ears flattened to the sides, perhaps with whiskers pulled back, are a sign of a fearful cat.

Tail signals

Tail signals are another means of feline communication: when the cat wags or swishes his tail, unlike in a dog this is not generally a sign of contentment. The more violent the swishing, the more the cat is excited or likely to act aggressively. A cat on the defensive will often bring his tail up and over in an arch, with the fur bristled to make it appear bigger. A tail held high with a slight forward/sideways bend at the tip is a common greeting signal to a friendly cat or human. When not being used for communication, the cat's tail reverts to its role in balancing the movements of the body in walking, running, jumping and climbing.

Helping people and cats with Bach remedies

Helping cats with Bach remedies is much, much more satisfying than helping humans! As any psychologist will tell you, humans can be tough to help. Sometimes they don't really want to be helped – they often resist getting better as they secretly or unconsciously relish the attention they get when they're depressed or miserable; at other times, people are unwilling to let go of an emotional 'crutch' that they've latched on to for support, such as alcohol or drugs, eating disorders or other types of behaviour. Humans with repressed emotional lives often recoil from confronting issues in their lives that they'd simply prefer not to think about – these can be things about themselves that they don't want to deal with, or aspects of their lives that are too frightening or painful to face up to. It's often easier for humans simply to go on repressing their pain, or redirecting their neuroses in ways that give them solace even though they may be harmful. So when humans are faced with a therapy like Bach flower remedies that offer them the potential for freedom from all these problems, which can start the process of loosening the knots that have gained a stranglehold on their personality, they may sometimes shy away. These emotional problems are often disguised as scepticism: it's easier to say 'I don't believe in that stuff' than it is to admit 'I'm terrified of throwing my crutch away'.

When it comes to helping an animal such as a cat, we can breathe a big sigh of relief, because animals present no such difficulties. Left to their own devices, cats are psychologically far healthier than most of us humans! Perhaps because they're so much closer to nature already, and have such a 'head start' on us, they often tend to respond faster and better to the remedies than humans do. A cat's recovery from emotional stress or psychological pain is a much more simple and uncomplicated business, and anyone who has ever helped a cat with Bach remedies can testify to the great satisfaction it brings to watch them changing, softening, losing their fear, regaining trust, learning to leave behind a difficult past and reclaiming their natural state of contentedness and vitality. You never lose the sense of wonder that comes with being able to help alleviate a cat's, or any animal's, emotional suffering with flower remedies.

Key areas for feline Bach flower therapy

There are several basic key areas of Bach flower therapy for cats and other animals. These are typical types of negative emotional/psychological states, situations or problems that seem to come up again and again and are the basis for much of feline Bach therapy.

Effects of past trauma

This is one of the most important areas of animal flower therapy, helping cats that have been adversely and lastingly affected by traumatic psychological experiences (or physical trauma for that matter) insofar as it may involve great fear). Examples of what can constitute a past trauma include:

- Acute moments of fear, terror, pain, beatings, attacks from people or other animals such as other cats, dogs or (occasionally) foxes.

- Chronic situations that the cat has had to endure, such as periods of ongoing cruelty from previous owners, daily extreme stress from being ill-treated, starved or confined.

- Any other kind of accident, shock, period of stress or other unpleasant incident.

Any cat that has been exposed to these kinds of stimuli for any length of time can be seriously affected and suffer terrible ongoing mental stress as a result. Animal rescue workers, who deal daily with cruelty cases and animals that have been psychologically abused, are all too aware of the suffering caused to their charges, and the tendency for a badly frightened, traumatised animal to fall physically ill in just the same way as an emotionally traumatised human being can decline into poor health. Even with medical care and a good diet, many of these animals remain unhealthy until their fears, stress and past traumas are helped. Bach flower remedies are an ideal way of helping to achieve this. What the Bach flower remedies, notably Star of Bethlehem, are uniquely able to do is to target the underlying traumatic experience, the cause of the problem, even if it happened a long time previously. The remedies can also be used to address the problems that have been created by the traumatic experience, which are the symptoms we see in the cat's behaviour telling us that all isn't well. These can be things such as fear, nervousness, lack of confidence, dislike of men, and so on.

Fears and anxiety

Fear or anxiety, in its various forms, is one of the biggest problems suffered by cats. As with most types of animal, the cat's options in a frightening situation are basically twofold: he can either run away or he can defend himself using aggression. Given the chance, a cat will generally prefer to run and take cover in some safe place, and may be extremely unwilling to emerge even if coaxed with treats. Failing the 'flight' option, a cat may have to resort to defensive aggression: howling, bristling, spitting, swiping and baring teeth. In some cases, cats do neither of these things. Instead, crouching very still, they avoid eye contact and simply seem to 'shut down' in the face of the frightening stimulus. This type of helpless behaviour is sometimes seen in extremely traumatised cats, for instance cats from a 'rescue' background. Whatever the cause of the fearfulness or the cat's reaction to it, Bach flower remedies have a major role to play in helping to reduce this enormous problem and we will be examining this in more detail later in the book.

Stress

Care and prevention of stress reactions is another important area in animal Bach flower therapy. Although their emotional lives may not be as complex as ours in some ways, they are just as capable of becoming stressed, anxious, confused, depressed and insecure. Managing stress levels for all animals will help to keep their immune system in good shape and help prevent the onset of illness – or if it does strike, it can help their system to deal with it more efficiently. Feline stress can show up in a number of ways:

- **Restless behaviour:** The cat may chase his tail, pace up and down or round and round, and never seem to relax.

- **Fur pulling and self-mutilation:** As a way to try to compensate for the stress, some cats can develop various obsessive-compulsive behaviours including fur-pulling and self- mutilation. This seems to occur mainly in certain specific breeds, notably the Burmese. Some behaviourists state that such behaviour is simply inherited; however in many cases it appears related to stress, boredom, or lack of mental stimulation, most often seen in cats kept confined indoors.

- **Tension in muscles:** The whole body may feel stiff and the cat's gait can be awkward. Stiffness like this can result from a state of prolonged mental stress. When the stress and mental tension is eased, there can be a relaxing of the physical level soon afterwards.

- **Cat seems to be depressed:** A depressed cat will tend to have little energy and appear to have lost his 'vital spark'. Always check with the vet to make sure nothing is physically wrong with the cat. It's often the case that such a cat will have nothing wrong with him physically/ medically, but just feels emotionally low and depressed.

- **Spraying and destructiveness in the home:** Stressed cats may cause havoc in the home by repeatedly scent-marking the furniture and/or clawing walls, curtains and so on. In a great many cases this behaviour is simply an expression of the cat's boredom and frustration at being excessively confined indoors.

- **Tendency to suffer from allergies:** Cats that have suffered a lot of stress over a long period can suffer a weakening of their immune system and be prone to allergies. If your cat has allergies it doesn't necessarily mean he's suffering from stress, but this is one possible factor.

- **Poor coat condition:** Patchy, matted, dry, shedding coats, or coats that lack lustre and vitality, may be signs of stress.

They could also be signs of physical illness, so always check this isn't the case.

- **Digestive or bowel problems:** Just like humans, there are cases where certain cats (often rescues) suffer from long-term stomach problems, e.g. colitis, due to past or present stress. Using Bach remedies is an important part of solving these problems, although because the stress has now had this chronic physical effect it may be necessary to use other therapies. Other complementary therapies, such as homeopathy and magnet therapy, have been known to help with these problems.

Stress and the overcrowding problem

In urban areas, one of the great sources of stress for cats is over-crowding, with too many cats occupying too many intersecting territories. Cats evolved to live spread out, each with their own personal space. A certain minimum of uncrowded private territory is required in order for cats to enjoy the stress-free and stimulating life that nature intended. Sadly, the enormous popularity of the cat as a pet has meant that humans interfere with this delicate social structure: because of us, there are simply too many of them living too close together. While certain Bach remedies can help to compensate for those individual cats who are affected by this and become stressed, insecure or fearful, the onus is on our human society to recognise and respect the nature and culture of the cat generally.

Physical stress-related conditions

The question of treating stress-related or emotional problems that have had an effect on the physical body is a complex issue. Dr Bach claimed in his writings that treating the mental/emotional problem behind the physical illness was enough to cure the physical illness. This was what he meant when he said we should 'treat the person, not the disease'.

Was Dr Bach right about this? In lighter cases, when stress is causing minor physical problems that have not been there for very long, there's no doubt that Bach remedies can have a very good indirect effect on the physical level. However, in more serious cases, such as chronic stomach ulcers that have their roots in stress, Bach remedies can heal the mental/emotional or stress related problems but have often not been shown to cure the chronic physical illness. Cats that suffer prolonged or extreme stress, such as rescue cats that may have been beaten or suffered cruel treatment, and then go on to suffer immune system breakdown and/or chronic physical disease, can benefit from Bach flower therapy for their emotional and behavioural problems, but the remedies should not be relied on to treat the physical illnesses arising from their past stresses. Nonetheless, the Bach remedies remain a very important complementary part of the cat's overall care program.

Other areas of Bach therapy for cats:

'Sponge' effect

Sponge effect gets its name from the fact that cats can soak up like a sponge the emotional negativity of the people they live with. This phenomenon can potentially affect any intelligent species that lives with humans, but in practice it tends to be much less of a problem for cats than it is for dogs, for the reason that cats can generally distance themselves more easily from the source of the stress. However, a cat that is confined indoors will potentially be more susceptible to this problem, just like a dog. Certain breeds like the Burman and the Siamese, whose owners often tend to keep them inside for their own reasons, may be more vulnerable. Certain flower remedies, notably Bach's Walnut, have the ability to offer protection against negative atmospheres by reducing the cat's sensitivity to them. The negative influences that most affect cats are the emotional energies projected by unhappy or angry, bitter people – such as the atmosphere you can 'cut with a knife' that lingers in the homes of argumentative families and people suffering from prolonged stress. Flower remedies can be extremely useful to help the people too, for their own sake and for the sake of the cats who have to live with them!

Recuperation from illness

This is another major area for this therapy. Whether an animal is receiving conventional medication, homeopathy or some other therapy, Bach flower therapy is of great benefit as an adjunct therapy helping the animal to cope and maintain vital energy over a long period of time. In many cases, flower remedies have been used as a 'pick me up' for animals that might not recover after an operation when their vital energy has dipped very low. Older cats are especially prone to long-drawn out recoveries from illness, and the psychological boost offered by certain Bach remedies can be extremely important to help them back on their feet. One of the real virtues of these remedies is that they can be given alongside any type of medication, and so are ideally suited to playing a complementary role for sick or recuperating animals.

Pet bereavement

This is another important area of use for the Bach remedies, which we'll return to in more detail later in the book. Humans and cats can often be equally affected by the death of a companion. Some cats will go into a state of deep depression after losing a friend (sometimes an owner, though more usually another cat). Most people who have had cats are all too familiar with the sense of loss when one dies. Certain Bach remedies are very important in helping ease the pain of pet loss.

When Bach remedies might not be the best or only approach

It's important to realise that many feline behavioural problems may have a variety of causes. If, for instance, a cat has become aggressive or depressed, it may be a mistake to judge this purely as an emotional or psychological problem – he could be in pain, or be suffering from some other medical disorder whose treatment lies outside the jurisdiction, or effective range, of Bach flower therapy. If a cat is behaving out of character, before thinking about Bach flower therapy always make sure that there's nothing medically wrong with the cat that could be distressing him, by checking with the vet. Flower remedies can help to alleviate mental stress associated with pain or illness, but aren't the appropriate treatment for the pain or illness itself. If it turns out that the cat is ill or in pain, we can use Bach remedies to help together with what the vet does.

Chapter Three

The 38 Remedies

In this main section of the book we're going to take a guided tour of the whole collection of remedies created by Dr Bach. To help gain an authentic historical flavour of Bach's work, the remedies are examined in the order he developed them.

Each remedy is examined from a human, and then a feline perspective. This not only allows us to develop a closer feeling for the use of each remedy, it also gives interesting insights into some of the similarities and differences in the ways that humans and cats think, feel and perceive the world about them. It's always important to bear in mind that many of the emotional and psychological states that occur in humans are not found in cats, or are experienced and expressed in a different way by the cat. One of the dangers of interpreting the uses of Bach remedies for cats is to fall into the trap of anthropomorphic thinking, that is, to ascribe human characteristics to animals. Cats are actually very lucky that they aren't as crazy as humans! This means that, although each and every Bach remedy has a potential use within feline care, some of the Bach flower remedies are less frequently used for animals than for people. In this section, Bach remedies that are found to be the most often needed and used for cats (and other animals) are marked with an asterisk (*).

Although we'll be looking at the remedies individually, the reader should be aware from the start that the best results with this therapy are often obtained when using remedies in combination with one another. It's possible to combine up to 8 or so Bach remedies, addressing different elements or 'angles' of a problem. Again, we'll be learning more about this later in the book. In the meantime, a good knowledge of each individual remedy will help you to create effective combinations later on.

IMPATIENS*

Latin name:	Impatiens glandulifera
Dr Bach's words:	'Those who are quick in thought and action and wish all things to be done without hesitation and delay. When ill they are anxious for a hasty recovery'
Keynotes:	**Impatience, frustration, pressure, stress**
Goal of therapy:	**To restore a sense of relaxation and serenity**

Impatiens for People: The very first remedy Dr Bach developed is also one of the most important. Impatiens is a remedy for an impatient, pressing, driving state of mind: a state of tension. The mind is wound-up, with a sense of urgency to move fast and 'get things done'. Such people may regard themselves as the leader in any situation – and in fact quite often the Impatiens 'type' of person is very capable and quick-thinking. The remedy is needed when natural skill and leadership tend to border over into ruthlessness, intolerance, anger, frustration, dissatisfaction and irritability – all of which take their toll and make it hard for the person to gain inner peace. The state doesn't switch off when the person is off-duty, either, but stays in the mind, gnawing away constantly. The goal of the remedy is to help give inner peace and freedom from restless pressure and agitation.

Impatiens for Cats: If we think about it, the use of Impatiens basically boils down to how we respond to, and deal with, stress. Cats by nature are very patient animals, and they don't normally need a remedy like Impatiens to help with impatient or demanding character traits of this kind as a human might. However, the key thing here is the ability of the Impatiens remedy to help relax the mind and reduce stress, and as under certain circumstances cats are very susceptible to mental stress, it's in this way that the remedy can help them most.

Any situation where a cat seems over-wrought, tense, worried, stressed, can call for the Impatiens remedy to bring greater calm. For instance it could be used to help soothe the mind of a cat that is recovering from illness or undergoing medical treatment, when he may feel irritable, restless and generally uptight. If a cat seems to have a 'highly-strung' temperament, Impatiens is one remedy that could be used to help reduce stress or tension levels. (It would be wise to check with a vet that this state of tension, if it's an ongoing thing, doesn't indicate some kind of medical issue such as a nagging pain or other source of discomfort.) It's also important, if a cat seems continually stressed, to try to identify what might be causing it, and to take whatever other measures are appropriate. For example, if a cat is under stress as a result of being confined indoors all the time, it would be wrong and unfair – not to mention ineffective – to try to rely on Impatiens as a remedy for this. Cats should, as far as possible, be allowed to express their natural need to roam freely over their personal territory and their wider range.

MIMULUS*

Latin Name:	Mimulus Guttatus
Dr Bach's words:	'Fear of accidents, of unknown things, of people, of strangers, of crowds, of being alone, of the dark… the fears of everyday life'
Keynotes:	**General fears and anxiety, nervousness**
Goal of therapy:	**To restore confidence and calm**

Mimulus for People: The Mimulus remedy is for all those everyday fears, for being anxious in regard to something concrete – for humans this includes things such as a driving test or exam, or having to stand up in public and give a talk. Generally, Mimulus is indicated for anticipated fearful events, fears of known objects, people or situations. People chronically in need of Mimulus are often shy and retiring, may not openly share or express their fears, but are generally nervy and fearful and tend to lack a strong character.

Mimulus for Cats: The remedy is used much in the same way for cats as for people. Cats needing Mimulus will tend to be underconfident and have fears of certain things, perhaps situations where they feel scared and vulnerable. The positive effect of Mimulus on cats is to encourage greater confidence and help them to deal with situations better.

Mimulus is a very commonly used remedy for cats, as many of their problems are related to fear, anxiety and nervousness. Fear of a more acute or extreme type, which could be described as a state of terror, calls for a different Bach remedy, Rock Rose. This can be given in addition to Mimulus, or perhaps simply instead of it. Mimulus may help with quite severe fears in cats, but tends to work more slowly than Rock Rose, because it's dealing with less extreme, less sudden and less acute states of fear and anxiety.

Research has shown that a fear remedy like Mimulus tends to address the outer 'layer' of the cat's mental state, and while it can be very useful in helping with fears, if the fear stems from something like a past trauma (this could be anything from an attack by another cat, to having been injured by a car, to an experience of cruel treatment in the past) you may find that the best results will be obtained from combining the fear remedy with another that will act on the root of the trauma. For this, see Star of Bethlehem.

CLEMATIS*

Latin name:	Clematis vitalba
Dr Bach's words:	'Those who are dreamy, drowsy, not fully awake, not really happy in their present circumstances… in illness some make little or no effort to get well'
Keynotes:	**Indifference, boredom, detachment**
Goal of therapy:	**To restore focus, interest and concentration**

Clematis for People: Discovered not very long after Impatiens, Bach's Clematis is really the complete antithesis of the earlier remedy. While Impatiens helped with impatient, pressing states of mind, Clematis is a remedy that helps the opposite state, that of dreaminess and a sense of not being 'with it'. People needing Clematis are not fully grounded in the here and now. They are somehow detached, dreamy, disconnected, and may seem very distracted when you are talking to them. Sometimes they may long for better times; life in the present appears boring and unfulfilling. They may spend much time daydreaming, and suffer from sleepiness and a lack of mental alertness. The remedy helps to restore these, and also to help in stressful situations where people react by becoming slow-thinking and 'out of it'. This is the reason Clematis was included in the famous 'Rescue Remedy' emergency formula.

Clematis for Cats: We don't really know a great deal about what goes on in the inner mind of a cat. It would be easy to state that cats don't have romantic longings, have fantasies or spend time dreaming. However, some cats are observed to seem to live 'in their own world', as though disconnected from things around them – so who knows what thoughts might be going through their minds? Some cat owners claim that their cats make little noises and movements in their sleep that seem to suggest they are experiencing some form of dream. One Siamese owner reported to the authors that they have witnessed their cat waking up from an apparent nightmare in exactly the same way people do. If it's true that cats dream, we can only suppose it's a normal and harmless part of their life and not something they might need a remedy for. However, in certain cases, if a cat seems excessively dreamy while awake, or may be tending to withdraw into himself as a way of coping with stress, it could be time to think about offering some gentle help. Here, Clematis would be good to team up with a remedy like Impatiens, as well as another we haven't looked at yet, Wild Rose. If the dreamy state were possibly connected to a past trauma of some kind – for instance if a rescue cat with an unknown past tended to withdraw a lot into himself, you might think of combining Clematis, Wild Rose and Star of Bethlehem. It would also be wise to have the cat seen by the vet, just to make sure as far as possible that there isn't some unseen medical cause behind the problem.

AGRIMONY*

Latin Name:	Agrimonia eupatoria
Dr Bach's words:	'People who love peace and are distressed by argument or quarrel, to avoid which they will agree to give up much'
Keynotes:	**Mental torture and worry, sensitivity to disturbances and disharmony**
Goal of therapy:	**To restore inner peace and tranquility**

Agrimony for People: Agrimony is a remedy that helps people who are very easily subjected to worries, discord, or commotion. They carry a burden of anxiety that becomes too much to bear if weighted by any additional pressure from the outside. However, rather than try to deal with the anxiety that is gnawing at them, they often try to hide or suppress it behind a veneer of false cheerfulness. This sometimes leads to a varying degree of dependence on alcohol or drugs. The kind of person who surprises all their friends and family by falling into a deep and sudden depression after years of seeming cheerful and happy, is a classic 'Agrimony type'. What the remedy does is to help free the mind from that inner pressure of anxiety. Sometimes trapped unconscious feelings are brought to the surface before being released. The person may go through a brief phase where one comes face-to-face with these upsetting emotions, but this temporary so-called 'healing crisis' should not be regarded as a negative thing but rather a cathartic and healthy experience.

Agrimony for Cats: Cats are very peace-loving creatures, and in their natural state they would suffer none of the psychological stress of living in a dysfunctional environment. Unfortunately, because we have brought this animal into the unnatural and problematic human world, they are often compelled to live with people who are unhappy and shout and argue with one another. Cats are very affected if they have to live in an atmosphere of conflict or quarrel. If unable to distance themselves physically by slipping out through a cat-flap or an open window, they will wait patiently for it to be over, trying to keep out of the way and feeling very stressed. If this situation happens often, it will become a source of chronic stress for the cat. The cat may become nervous and confused, or even quite depressed. Cats that suffer from this kind of stress can be helped with Agrimony, but it's also important for people to address their own emotional problems and think about the effect they are having on the animal.

Agrimony can help any cat suffering from stress, and as such it makes a good companion to the Bach remedy Impatiens. Another related remedy is Walnut, helping cats to deal with stressful outside influences. These three remedies in combination can be very helpful to ease the stress of situations like kenneling, confinement at the vet's, quarantine, introduction to a new household or any other experience that could be disquieting to them.

CHICORY*

Latin name:	Cichorium intybus
Dr Bach's words:	'Those who are very mindful of the needs of others; they tend to be over-full of care for children, relatives, friends, always finding something that should be put right'
Keynotes:	**Possessive or controlling hold over others**
Goal of therapy:	**Letting go, developing emotional independence**

Chicory for People: Chicory is a very powerful and important remedy for those who are possessive towards others, for those who try to bind others to them. The Chicory person needs the closeness of others for comfort and reassurance, which we all do; but they also have this need to influence and control. The Chicory person seeks affection, but is often very possessive in relationships with others, friends, family and children. They like to express their affection, but they also require a response from you. Without this response, they can withdraw and start pouting, and become offended. So there is a two-sided aspect to the Chicory state, which can alternate quite rapidly – there's the outgoing and expressive affectionate state, very giving and fussy; and there is the state of self-pity and withdrawal, looking for attention. In short, Chicory addresses the common human tendency to be self-centred, manipulative and controlling.

Chicory for Cats: Cats can become really expert at manipulating their owners to gain attention. Attention-seeking cats are really at the opposite end of the spectrum from the traditional concept of the aloof, disdainful cat who wouldn't lower himself to spend time with people! Cats may develop attention-seeking tendencies due to being taken from their mothers too early, or perhaps being bottle-fed by humans at a very young age. Others develop a certain emotional neediness after an illness, having been very reliant on people for their care during that time. Signs of this emotional dependency include 'kittenish' behaviour towards humans, mewing and following them around, needing to be with them constantly. These cats can become chronic attention-seekers, and the behaviour can get quite out of hand – cats will even learn to get attention by ripping the furniture or knocking things off tables and shelves just to distract you!

It's important for owners to recognise the ways in which it's all too easy to encourage attention-seeking behaviour. People can be flattered by the attentions of an emotionally needy cat and return the affection without realising that they're really just compounding the problem. If you have a cat that seeks your attention in other ways, for instance by being destructive, shouting or reprimanding him might be the very thing he's looking for! In such cases it would be better to try to ignore the behaviour, and in so doing withdraw the reward that the cat receives for his actions.

Chicory can help in this process, by acting to reduce the cat's urgent need to gain your attention. The remedy helps the cat to achieve greater emotional independence. There have been cases where Chicory alone was able to stop the attention-seeking behaviour; in other cases the remedy's action needs to be backed up by actively paying attention to teaching the cat new habits.

Attention-seeking can also be a sign that a cat is bored and under-stimulated. Always make sure that cats are as free as possible to explore their world and exercise their innate feline instincts.

VERVAIN

Latin name:	Verbena officinalis
Dr Bach's words:	'They have a great wish to convert all around them to their own views of life'
Keynotes:	**Overenthusiasm, excessive exuberance, 'in your face'**
Goal of therapy:	**To restore calm, composure and sedate behaviour**

Vervain for People: According to Dr Bach's interpretation, the type of person needing Vervain often wants to convert others to their own view, to their own principles. Vervain is also a good remedy for an excessively exuberant, demonstrative and 'hyper' person.

Such people can expend huge amounts of energy when they constantly take centre stage in any social situation, talking a great deal, being very forceful with their opinions in an attempt to influence others, acting very enthusiastically towards people who agree with them. However, when they have burnt up all their energy with this hyper-exuberant behaviour, they can often withdraw into a state of exhausted tension, have angry outbursts or even become very depressed.

Vervain for Cats: Cats are most certainly not interested in trying to convert others to their ways! Where this remedy can help cats is in helping to reduce the drive of excess energy that can result in exuberance, hyperactivity and uncontrollable behaviour.

When a cat acts in an apparently hyperactive way, never stops running about and is virtually climbing the walls, we can try Vervain by all means but should not be too surprised if it doesn't work! There may be all sorts of factors involved, including diet (the cat may be receiving too much energy in his food) and training (the way that people are responding to his 'hyper' behaviour may be shaping his own responses). For instance, if the cat is getting rewarded by attention each time he jumps up, this is simply teaching him that all this is a great game and a fun way of becoming the centre of attention. We can't then expect a Bach remedy to 'switch off' what we have taught him is the desired way to act. All of these factors may need to be addressed as well as using this remedy. Using Vervain in conjunction with a re-training program, e.g. gently but firmly and consistently ignoring the cat's 'hyper' behaviour, is likely to bring better results than relying on the remedy alone.

Especially in younger cats, displays of exuberance can often simply be a perfectly normal expression of their overflowing youthful energy. In such cases, giving Vervain cannot do any harm but is unlikely to make any difference!

If a cat starts suddenly displaying strangely overactive behaviour, and especially if he starts yowling day and night, it would be very wise to have a veterinary surgeon carry out tests for hyperthyroidism. This fairly common condition can cause behavioural changes. In such cases, Vervain may well work to complement the treatment prescribed by the vet.

CENTAURY

Latin Name:	Centaurium umbellatum
Dr Bach's words:	'Kind, quiet people who are over-anxious to serve others... they become more servants than willing helpers, do more than their own share of the work, and may neglect their own particular mission in life'
Keynotes:	**Weakness, too willing servitor, the 'doormat'**
Goal of therapy:	**To restore greater assertiveness and confidence**

Centaury for People: Centaury is what could be called the 'doormat' remedy. The remedy helps people with an underconfident and vulnerable state of mind where they feel they have to allow everyone to dominate them. In the Centaury state one is terribly eager to please and serve others. This is no bad thing in itself, in fact a highly commendable trait – and Centauries are often really nice, sweet people with a heart of gold. But the problem centres on the person's difficulty in asserting themselves and stopping more forceful personalities from dominating them completely and taking them for granted. In short, Centaury is about empowerment: finding the inner strength needed to stand up for one's own freedom. Centaury doesn't take away the love of helping and serving others, it allows a person to find the right balance between giving to others and expecting something back in return.

Centaury for Cats: The main use for this remedy for cats is to help them develop greater confidence. In this way it is very closely related to the remedies Cerato and Larch.

A common feline behaviour problem is the issue of bullying over territory. Sadly, such situations are an extremely common reflection of the overcrowded cat populations in urban and suburban areas. Some cats are more naturally retiring by personality, whereas others are quick to intimidate. The bullies can become very tyrannical, driving the less confident cats away at every opportunity and making their lives very unhappy. The shy, retiring state can be thought of as a Centaury-type state, whilst the overdominant bully could be symbolised by the remedy Vine. Of course, it would be misleading to assert that by giving Centaury to the bullied cat and Vine to the bully, one could iron out the imbalance altogether in every case. However, the Centaury remedy has been known to help cats that tended to fall prey to 'bullies', giving them the extra courage to assert themselves and reclaim their right to a little private space where they can feel safe and secure. If a cat has become a little insecure as a result of his life experiences, other remedies may also be required to help – for instance Star of Bethlehem for the cat with a traumatic history.

CERATO

Latin name:	Ceratostigma willmottiana
Dr Bach's words:	'Those who have not sufficient confidence in themselves to make their own decisions. They constantly seek advice from others, and are often misguided'
Keynotes:	**Self-distrust, lack of self-belief**
Goal of therapy:	**To strengthen the personality**

Cerato for People: Cerato is a remedy for people who are hesitant with low self-confidence, who don't trust their own decisions. They will often be too reliant on other people's advice, unable to rely on their own judgement. For the same reason they often tend to be easily impressed by fads and trends, and are the kind of people to follow an opinion-leader without question. Cerato is often a good remedy for young people who have not yet developed a confident personality and may be very open to negative influences Cerato types are often shy by nature, lacking in forcefulness and confidence. The goal of the remedy is to help boost confidence and independence. Like Centaury it helps to foster a balanced degree of assertiveness, and like Chestnut Bud it helps to mature the personality.

Cerato for Cats: Cerato can be helpful to a young cat that lacks confidence and experience, for instance a kitten that has been taken away from his mother before she was able to teach him the important rules and 'facts of life' that a cat needs to know. This remedy can help the cat to gain more confidence in our confusing and alien human world. Cerato can help them to become surer of themselves. Another important remedy for helping cats with a lack of confidence is Larch.

SCLERANTHUS

Latin name:	Scleranthus annuus
Dr Bach's words:	'Those who suffer much from being unable to decide between two things, first one seeming right then the other'
Keynotes:	**Indecisiveness, vacillation between options**
Goal of therapy:	**To restore decisive balance, clarity and focus**

Scleranthus for People: The classic use of Scleranthus in people is in helping with choices and decision-making. People needing this remedy often have trouble making up their mind between different options. There is always vacillation, or swaying, in the negative Scleranthus state. This would be the sort of person who simply can't decide whether to go to Place A or Place B for their holiday and would sit there with a brochure in each hand, staring first at one and then at the other, would decide on A and start making arrangements for that, and then would change their decision and go for B, and then would change back again any number of times. Then, having travelled to Place B and sitting in their hotel room, their thoughts would start turning fretfully to what it would have been like to visit Place A instead! This chronic difficulty in deciding on a path and sticking to it can give rise to feelings of dissatisfaction, restlessness and unhappiness. Scleranthus can help the sufferer develop a more decisive and confident perspective that will improve their life generally.

Scleranthus for Cats: This is one of those cases where the uses of the remedy are a little different than for people. Cats generally don't suffer from indecisiveness. They're quick at making decisions once they understand the options facing them. For instance, if there's food involved and the cat works out the best and fastest way of getting it, their decision-making will be very quick indeed! Likewise, if something frightens a cat his decision to react accordingly will be instantaneous and logical: run away if possible, or stand and fight if flight isn't an option.

Thus, Scleranthus isn't so much indicated for indecisiveness in cats, but more for other types of vacillation. There have been reported cases of Scleranthus helping cats with physical problems that echo the Scleranthus 'swaying' tendency: these are problems such as hormonal swings, such as false pregnancies in cats. These are imbalances where a queen will go through all the motions of pregnancy even though not actually pregnant. She may show strange, unsettled behaviours, irritable one minute and normal the next. Scleranthus may be able to help settle these moods down.

The remedy has also been reported useful for car sickness in some cats, nausea caused by irregular motion. This may be due to some subtle inner balancing action that the remedy is capable of, although this is still unknown in neuroscience. Note: in some cases cats are sick in cars due to stress and nervousness, so other remedies should also be taken into account (such as Mimulus, Rock Rose and Impatiens) depending on the situation and the individual cat. When a cat is sick in the car due to a past trauma related to car travel, another important remedy is Star of Bethlehem.

WATER VIOLET*

Latin name:	Hottonia palustris
Dr Bach's words:	'For those who in health or illness like to be alone… they are aloof, leave people alone and go their own way'
Keynotes:	**Pride, aloofness, separation from others**
Goal of therapy:	**To restore a sense of social togetherness**

Water Violet for People: Water Violet is for people who deliberately keep away from others, often because they feel superior and are reluctant to associate with them or be on the same level as them. Dr Bach noticed that Water Violet types are often very clever and talented. They may feel special or more accomplished than other people, and this talent gives them a sense of being elevated above the rest of society. But hidden behind this veneer of great self-confidence there is often a painful sense of loneliness that stems from their inability to reach out to others and feel part of a warm social togetherness. The goal of this remedy is to help melt away the barriers and allow the person to meet with others on a more equal level.

Water Violet for Cats: It's easy to be misled by the keynotes of this remedy with regard to cats. Due to the popular conception of the cat as a proud, aloof, sometimes even disdainful creature, it might be possible to imagine that Water Violet could be used to help iron out these traits. However, this is missing the main point. The apparent 'pride' and 'aloofness' of cats isn't a sign of anything wrong with them – it isn't an emotional imbalance or a manifestation of repressed insecurity. It's simply a normal part of being a cat. As humans we tend to want to judge things from a human standpoint, and one of the problems associated with this is the anthropomorphic interpretation we sometimes place on animal behaviour and character. Our traditional portrayal of the cat as 'proud and aloof' probably accounts for why some people so strongly mistrust and dislike cats. But it's very unfair on the animal! Cats are neither 'proud' nor 'aloof'. They're just cats.

However, this isn't to say that Water Violet has no use in helping cats. The Water Violet state can exist in cats, though it's less complex than in humans. With cats, this remedy is helpful in helping to re-create social harmony. Cats are not as group-orientated as dogs, but nonetheless they can function very well on the periphery of a social group, tolerating the presence of others, even deriving a quiet comfort from the sense of unity. If for some reason a cat has problems adapting to this role, or seems completely unable to tolerate even the most passive membership of the social group, it could be a call for Water Violet to help deal with whatever underlying insecurity is causing this unease. The cat may have had bad experiences with people or other animals in the past, and as a result may have problems with trust. Water Violet could work well alongside remedies such as Star of Bethlehem, Mimulus and Larch in such a case. Cats that have been undersocialised may benefit from the remedy, helping them to develop a greater tolerance of humans. Rescue cats may require help to 'soften' their attitude to the social group. Likewise, when introducing new animals to the home, Water Violet can help to promote a sense of harmony between them. Another useful remedy in this role would be Walnut.

GENTIAN

Latin name:	Gentiana amarella
Dr Bach's words:	'Those who are easily discouraged. They may be progressing well in illness, or in the affairs of daily life, but any small delay or hindrance of progress causes doubt and soon disheartens them'
Keynotes:	**Doubt and discouragement**
Goal of therapy:	**To restore drive, determination and progress**

Gentian for People: Gentian is a remedy that works well when we lose faith or determination after a setback, or if things seem not to improve despite all our efforts. The negative Gentian state that comes on is a very deep sense of futility, with the belief that nothing we can do in life will ever succeed or get us anywhere. This negative attitude allows us to give up very easily in the face of even the slightest challenge. The remedy helps the person to develop greater optimism and faith, to find the strength inside them to face these challenges and develop greater stamina of the personality. The remedy is also important in states of physical illness when the person has little faith in their recovery or has doubts about the slow process of getting better. Helping to restore a positive attitude will have a beneficial effect on physical health as well, helping to promote a speedier and more complete recovery. This is another example of Dr Bach's ideas about a positive state of mind affecting the state of physical health.

Gentian helps to promote the determination we need to overcome adversity. This is nicely illustrated by an old historical story about Robert the Bruce, a Scottish warrior who fought for freedom and independence in medieval times. Hiding in a cave from English soldiers after losing a battle, Bruce felt utterly defeated. Then he saw a spider making a web on the wet cave wall. He watched how it kept falling but was never discouraged. Eventually it succeeded, after many failures to build its web in such a place. Bruce was very inspired by this. He decided that 'if at first you don't succeed, try, and try again'. This gave him the strength to overcome his pessimism and lead his armies to victory. Gentian has the same lesson to teach us.

Gentian for Cats: Cats, under normal circumstances, are rather similar to Bruce's spider: very resilient and not easily discouraged by challenges. However, Gentian can be very useful to a cat that has lost his vitality and drive, for instance in illness where it can help a cat that seems to be giving in to his ailment and not recovering well. It's a very good remedy to use during a cat's convalescence or at any time during his life when he needs support and strength.

Gentian is sometimes recommended for cats and other animals that lose their appetite or suddenly become despondent. While there's no harm in considering the use of this remedy, and always check with a vet in case this change in the animal's behaviour might indicate a medical problem. If it should turn out that medical treatment is needed, Gentian is one of the Bach remedies that could be used to help the animal through the process.

ROCK ROSE*

Latin Name: Helianthemum nummularium

Dr Bach's words: 'This is the remedy for cases when there appears no hope. In accidents or sudden illness, where the patient is very frightened or terrified, or if the condition is serious enough to cause great fear to those around.'

Keynotes: **Acute fear/terror**

Goal of therapy: **To restore courage and calm**

Rock Rose for People: The Rock Rose remedy was discovered for acute states of extreme fear and terror and their after-effects. During an acute state of terror there may be feelings of great danger, perhaps a fear of imminent death or injury, a great deal of mental turmoil and sometimes an overwhelming urge to run away. There is also a more chronic state of terror, where people feel constantly threatened, nervous and jittery. This kind of fear is distinct from the less extreme Mimulus type of anxiety, although in fact both of these fear remedies can be used together to 'cover' a fear problem from different 'angles' at once. The goal of the Rock Rose remedy is to promote courage, self control, and true heroism.

Rock Rose for Cats: Cats are just as capable as we are of feeling fear, both of the everyday anxiety kind (Mimulus) and of the more pressing, terrifying kind. Rock Rose can help them with great fear, terror and its after-effects. It can also help with chronic states of fearful anxiety, often seen in cats that have been beaten or badly looked after. Cats in this state lack confidence and show through their body language that they are very unhappy. Rock Rose is one of the remedies, together with others like Mimulus, Wild Rose, Star of Bethlehem, that can be considered in these circumstances. In acute situations, such as trying to calm down a cat that has been in an accident while waiting for the vet to arrive, Rock Rose has often been used effectively, for instance by adding a few drops to some water and moistening the cat's lips or temples.

Please note: *Never* put a glass dropper in a cat's mouth, and especially not if the cat is in a state of nervous agitation or panic.

GORSE*

Latin name:	Ulex europaeus
Dr Bach's words:	'Very great hopelessness, they have given up belief that more can be done for them'
Keynotes:	**Hopelessness, apathy and despair**
Goal of therapy:	**To restore hope and the will to go on**

Gorse for People: Gorse is for very deep and powerful emotional states of hopelessness bordering on despair: a feeling of black gloom and resignation, with all hope gone. This state of mind can come on after a personal tragedy or major blow, and persist for a long time. Physically, the person may lose vitality and their incentive to live, which is a dangerous state in sickness and can lead to a rapid decline. Gorse can lift the spirits and facilitate a new, more inspiring outlook into the beyond. It's a very useful remedy also for bereavement, where grief turns to bitter nihilism.

Gorse for Cats: These are emotional states that cats can fall into just the same as humans. Gorse has helped many cats suffering from deep gloom, depression and despair. They become shut off from the light, lose their will to live and survive, and can easily die if something isn't done to help them. A cat may shut down and go into this state after a loss of an owner, or if his life suddenly changes and he loses all the things that have brought comfort. Older cats may come to need this remedy, or cats that have suffered a traumatic experience from which they have trouble recovering psychologically. It's heartbreaking to see a cat fall into an emotional state where he doesn't care if he survives; but it's a very joyous experience to see such a cat respond to a remedy like Gorse. It's as though the light has returned, and the cat fills with the strength to go on. Gorse is a very important remedy, perhaps one of the most important.

OAK*

Latin name:	Quercus robur
Dr Bach's words:	'For those who are struggling and fighting strongly to get well... they will fight on against great difficulties, without loss of hope or effort'
Keynotes:	**Despondency from weakening resistance**
Goal of therapy:	**To restore reserves of energy and endurance**

Oak for People: Oak is a remedy able to give strength to people who, despite their efforts to overcome difficulties, are losing their resistance. This may be in a situation of illness, where extra strength is needed to overcome depletion and weakness; or it may apply to situations in life where circumstances, challenges or periods of hardship can affect our emotional strength.

There is a type of person who will display heroic feats of willpower, stoic determination to go on with their duties despite personal hardship and severity. As long as things go well for them, they can turn a blind eye to the pain they make themselves suffer; but as their reserves begin to dwindle – and we all have a breaking-point – setbacks and failures take their toll and feelings of futility and despondency quickly set in. Here, the Oak remedy can help them in two ways, by giving them access to fresh reserves of inner strength and also by helping them to relax their dedication to their duties and take some time to look after themselves more. This remedy works well with others such as Hornbeam and Olive, which both can help to refresh our inner reserves of strength.

Oak for Cats: Where Oak can help cats is in helping with a weakened 'vital force'. Cats, just like humans, can suffer a loss of loss of energy and vitality as a result of a long struggle or period of deprivation. This could be a crippling illness, or a period of maltreatment or neglect. Oak can be useful in helping to rekindle vital energies and enthusiasm for life. It can be very important to use in cases where cats are undergoing veterinary treatment, to help support their recovery. Cats can sometimes seem to 'shut down' emotionally as a result of a severe illness or trauma, and here Oak together with Bach remedies Gorse and Wild Rose can really help. All these remedies can help a cat to muster his strength in difficult times.

HEATHER

Latin name: Calluna vulgaris

Dr Bach's words: 'Those who are always seeking the companionship of anyone who may be available... they are very unhappy if they have to be left alone for any length of time'

Keynotes: **Self-preoccupation**

Goal of therapy: **To promote emotional independence**

Heather for People: Heather helps where the sufferer has problems connecting properly with others. You could describe the classic Heather state as 'unable to receive incoming calls'. People needing this remedy tend to be strongly self-centred and very absorbed with their own life and problems. They may feel a powerful urge to share these problems with others, in an attempt to gain attention, sympathy, or companionship. They are often very talkative, and often the listener finds themselves held there pinned, after a while probably wishing they could get away but also probably feeling guilty for wishing so! Should the listener try to bring up the issue of their own problems, the Heather type doesn't hear or doesn't connect, as they are just too preoccupied with themselves. While Heather-type behaviour may seem annoying and selfish, in many cases the only way a lonely, scared and insecure person can come to feel supported and understood. The saddest thing for them is that their way of forcing themselves on others can often have the opposite effect of driving those people away from them.

Heather for Cats: The essence of the Heather state in a person is mental tension with regard to their own situation and the need to express unhappiness. Cats can need Heather too, but the way they express their need is much less neurotic and complicated.

The Heather state in a cat is a little like the Chicory state. Cats can sometimes feel very 'left out' of our activities, and will attempt to redress the balance by gaining attention. They can be very persistent, and may develop a whole range of behaviours designed to gain your attention by flattery or by driving you wild with annoyance! These problems are often compounded by owners who have inadvertently trained the cat to think that by acting this way they can be rewarded. Heather can't retrain the cat to think differently, but can help to reduce the mental stress and desire for attention. It's then up to the owner to teach the cat that those attention-seeking behaviours aren't going to work any more!

ROCK WATER

Latin name:	'Aqua petra'
Dr Bach's words:	'Those who are very strict in their way of living; they deny themselves many of the joys and pleasures of life because they consider it might interfere with their work'
Keynotes:	**Mental rigidity, fixed habits**
Goal of therapy:	**Learning new ways and a flexible attitude**

Rock Water for People: Rock Water is interesting because out of all Dr Bach's remedies it's the only one not prepared from a flower! Dr Bach made this remedy from a source of spring water believed to have natural healing properties.

People in need of the Rock Water remedy have a particular tendency to be very self-controlling. They need to master themselves and overcome what they see as any adverse tendencies within themselves. In theory, this could be an admirable pursuit – but the Rock Water state is out of balance, because it becomes a self-punitive one. These people become their own 'army officer'; the so-called adverse tendencies they identify within themselves include desires, longings, vital needs, normal human emotions. They suppress these things and feel themselves to be very strong and very admirable; they are proud of the effort they have made. Rock Water people, in their sense of having accomplished something really special, often want to inspire others to follow their example. They may intimidate others, sometimes alienating them but also sometimes confusing and brainwashing them, while they themselves suffer a lot of emotional strain from their self-imposed regime. The goal of the remedy is to help the person ease up on themselves, while at the same time acting with more kindness to those around.

Rock Water for Cats: Thankfully for cats, once again their simpler psychology allows them to avoid getting into such a mess as a human! Where we see the Rock Water state in a cat, it's in a much less complex and neurotic form. Cats don't feel any desire to punish themselves, deny themselves the good things in life; they don't have any interest in setting a moral example or showing everyone how wonderful they are! Nor have they any interest in trying to convert you to the way they want to live. Cats simply are. And we humans have a lot to learn from them!

Where Rock Water can help cats is in helping them with states of mental rigidity. The remedy can help a training programme to work better by helping the cat to develop a more flexible attitude towards new ideas – common examples would be teaching a cat to use a cat flap, or introducing a cat to a litter tray for the first time. In any situation where old habits need to give way to new ones, there is a role for Rock Water in helping to soften rigid established patterns and create new pathways.

VINE*

Latin name:	Vitis vinifera
Dr Bach's words:	'Very capable people, certain of their own ability, confident of success. Being so assured, they think that it would be for the benefit of others if they could be persuaded to do things as they themselves do, or as they are certain is right'
Keynotes:	**Domination of others**
Goal of therapy:	**To mellow over-assertive behaviour**

Vine for People: The mental/emotional state helped by the remedy is one of domination and control. Vine 'types', rather like Impatiens types but more forceful, are often convinced of their leadership qualities and very frequently assume control over others whether or not these others are happy about it. They tend to disregard people's opinions and wishes in an overbearing way. In extreme cases, this tendency towards controlling behaviour may lead to ruthlessness or even violence as a means of staying in charge. There are also the less overtly dominant Vine types who tend to use manipulation, flattery and other tricks to help them achieve their ends. They can seem very friendly and earnest, but are no less dominating – as William Shakespeare wrote, 'a man can smile, and smile, and be a villain'. The former more dictatorial state often emerges when the latter has failed. However their tendencies show themselves, these people will be very goal-orientated and lacking in compassion for others. The Vine remedy helps them to regain compassion, essentially by relieving the deep fear that drives them.

Vine for Cats: This remedy can help to mellow extremes of dominant or over-assertive behaviour in cats. These behaviours, which can include bullying or sometimes aggressive behaviour, are often inappropriate expressions of natural dominant behaviour. Cats don't have such a clear-cut dominance hierarchy as dogs, but nonetheless 'power struggles' are quite common between them. Whilst dogs are mainly concerned with the responsibility of leading the pack for the good of the collective, cats are more concerned with the important business of claiming and maintaining a territory of their own. The growth of the cat population in built-up areas does nothing to ease matters, and territorial disputes are very common, even inside the home if two or more cats have been brought to live together in close proximity. Vine can never erase a cat's natural territorial instincts, but what it can do is help to reduce the pressing need for one cat to constantly assert himself over another. Like Water Violet, Beech and Holly, it's a remedy that helps to promote social harmony, peace and tolerance.

OLIVE*

Latin name:	Olea europa
Dr Bach's words:	'Those who have suffered much mentally or physically and are so exhausted and weary that they feel they have no more strength to make any effort. Daily life is hard work for them, without pleasure'
Keynotes:	**Mental and physical weariness**
Goal of therapy:	**To restore energy and drive**

Olive for People: This remedy is for deep states of exhaustion, where people are badly in need of regeneration and extra reserves of energy. The Olive state is one where the person has reached their limits and are just too tired to go on, feeling burnt out. They may find themselves feeling unable to get excited about anything: life becomes dull and unrewarding and they may sink into sadness and apathy. The remedy helps to relieve the problem by promoting a renewal of energy and enthusiasm.

Olive for Cats: Olive works in the same way for cats as it does for humans. It can help to restore energy in cats suffering from physical and mental exhaustion after a period of hardship, stress or illness, making it a useful remedy with a diverse range of potential uses. It can be helpful for rescue cats, sick or recuperating cats, old cats or any cat that has been through a taxing experience and is suffering from loss of drive. Olive works very well together with Wild Rose for cats that seem to have given up the will to go on after a very difficult experience such as a period of illness.

WILD OAT

Latin name:	Bromus ramosus
Dr Bach's words:	'Those who have ambitions to do something of prominence in their life, who wish to have much experience, and to take life to the full'
Keynotes:	**Lack of motivation and incentive**
Goal of therapy:	**To catalyse, energise and move forward**

Wild Oat for People: People needing Wild Oat tend to feel unmotivated, stale and bored with their lives, feeling that they could be doing something more stimulating but often unaware how to find it or achieve it. They often don't have a calling, or they are unsure what it could be – they have trouble identifying a goal or path in their life. People needing this remedy often try several different paths but nothing seems quite right. They can become listless and frustrated, and life loses joy and sparkle for them. The remedy acts as a sort of 'rut-buster' that helps to restart their floundering system and motivates them to find a satisfying new direction, or else give a boost to an old one gone stale.

Wild Oat for Cats: Wild Oat is so well known as the 'career / life path remedy' that it's easy to get sidetracked by this view when it comes to considering its role in feline care. It would be absurd to suggest that Wild Oat could help a cat figure out what he wanted to do with his life! Cats don't have problems about their career path or what motivates them in life. As long as they have the basic needs of company, shelter and most importantly food, they are generally happy. Cats just want to be cats, and they need no remedies to help them achieve 'catness'.

What they do occasionally need, though, is a helping hand at times when they lack drive and energy in their lives. Essentially, Wild Oat's action is as a catalyst and energiser, helping to create new pathways for moving forward – and this is how to regard this remedy for the purposes of feline care. Dr Bach observed that giving this remedy could enhance the actions of other Bach flowers. He noticed that where a case was 'stuck' or there was lack of progress in treatment, adding Wild Oat to the chosen list of remedies could act to unblock the process. If, for instance, a cat was generally down and lacking in drive and energy, adding Wild Oat to a blend of remedies such as Oak, Olive, Hornbeam, Wild Rose and Gentian may help to create a more dynamic effect. Remember, though, always to have your cat checked by the vet if he shows a sudden drop in energy levels, vitality and joy of living. Should this turn out to have some medical cause, the Bach remedies can still be used alongside any other treatment.

Another important use of Wild Oat in feline care is in helping cats indirectly by making their owners happier and more satisfied with life. Having to live with someone who suffers from a negative Wild Oat state could be very stressful for a cat. If the person helped themselves with this or any other needed remedy, the benefits they felt would also act to reduce the 'sponge effect' or secondary stress felt by the cat.

CHERRY PLUM*

Latin name:	Prunus cerasifera
Dr Bach's words:	'Fear of the mind being over-strained, of reason giving way, of doing fearful and dreaded things… there comes the thought and impulse to do them'
Keynotes:	**Fear of losing mental balance**
Goal of therapy:	**To restore calm, balance and inner peace**

Cherry Plum for People: In the Cherry Plum state, the mind is overstrained and out of balance, with a sense of struggling against itself. A Cherry Plum state can come on during a period of stress, when we feel like cracking and may fall in a heap of tears or else have a fit of rage and smash something that we will regret later! Cherry Plum can be of use in nervousness, shyness, and stage fright, these being unwanted mental states where one tries to fight against oneself. Cherry Plum has also often helped more serious emotional states where sufferers feel severe internal pressure that influences their behaviour. It's an effective remedy where there is frightening loss of control, and some psychologists have used the remedy to help patients with self-destructive tendencies. Cherry Plum's goal is to reduce pressure from the unconscious, to give mental peace and relaxation.

Cherry Plum for Cats: Once again we see that, luckily for cats, they don't fall prey to the same depths of mental torment as humans. However, cats are capable, at a certain level, of experiencing mental/emotional stress that can push them over the edge. Cherry Plum helps cats suffering from extremes of stress that create erratic thought processes, hysterical or aggressive behaviour. The remedy can help to bring calm in frightening situations that threaten to tip the cat's mind into panic or loss of control.

ELM*

Latin name:	Ulmus procera
Dr Bach's words:	'At times there may be periods of depression when they feel that the task they have undertaken is too difficult, and not within the power of a human being'
Keynotes:	**Overwhelm, loss of will**
Goal of therapy:	**Ability to deal calmly with pressure**

Elm for People: Elm is for states of being overwhelmed and subdued by tasks, duties or responsibilities that seem to loom over us and appear irresolvable. The more we focus on the problem, the less we are able to focus on the solution: this becomes a vicious circle that may start a decline into great mental stress, even despair and despondency. It may be a sign that the sufferer has been working too hard and needs to rest; after a break the mind may perceive things differently. The goal of the Elm remedy is to help the mind to relax and step back from things and gain a fresher perspective. The remedy helps to organise the mind, to give it clarity and to allow a person to grow beyond their troubles.

Elm for Cats: Cats can become very overwhelmed and mentally stressed by too many impressions happening at once. They are perfectly adapted to the slower, more focused pace of nature, but our modern human society can be very bewildering to them. Cats that have to live in chaotic or stressful environments such as catteries or rescue centres can become confused and unhappy. Though of course we need to do everything possible to reduce the amount of stress a cat has to deal with, Elm can additionally help the cat by relaxing his mind in the face of all these potentially troubling impressions.

Similarly, Elm can also be very helpful in kitten socialisation, where young cats are introduced for the first time to the many things they have to learn to deal with in life. Giving Elm to the cat for a period of time can be a major help through this process, helping to prevent the youngster from becoming overwhelmed by all the new sense impressions such as rooms full of unknown people, the veterinary surgery, and meeting up with other animals. It's important that a young cat should make positive associations with all these things early in life, as a cat that is allowed to become frightened by early socialisation experiences will often grow up to become a nervous adult. Another important remedy to aid socialisation is Walnut, along with courage and confidence-giving remedies such as Larch, Mimulus and Cerato.

ASPEN*

Latin name:	Populus tremula
Dr Bach's words:	'Vague unknown fears, for which there can be given no explanation, no reason... yet the patient may be terrified of something terrible going to happen'
Keynotes:	**Fears of unclear or unconscious origin**
Goal of therapy:	**Confidence and courage**

Aspen for People: Aspen deals with a particular kind of fear that needs to be distinguished from Mimulus or Rock Rose-type fears. People in need of Aspen are fearful, often with a sense of hovering anxiety, an undercurrent of panic, but they have difficulty understanding the root of their fear. An Aspen-type fear is more mysterious than a simple fear of a thing, place, person, or experience. It's often linked to supernatural or metaphysical fears from the unconscious, or a deep psychological fear of the unknown that may be reflected in the person's dreams. Deep fears of the unknown, of the future, of what lies beyond death, are all glimpses of the workings of our unconscious mind. If we are unconsciously full of tension and anxiety, this will tend to filter through to the conscious mind as this nebulous, undefined Aspen-type nervousness. The remedy, then, addresses fears that we may not even be fully aware of consciously, helping to make life easier by relieving that inner burden.

Aspen for Cats: Cats normally will always have a clear idea what they are afraid of, and will generally behave accordingly. For instance if there is a certain person they fear, when that person comes into the room the cat is likely to start acting fearfully. Animals don't, as far as we know, have the same kind of unconscious or metaphysical fears that we more complex humans have. These facts tend to indicate that we are less likely to see the classic Aspen-type fears affecting cats.

However, this doesn't mean that Aspen cannot be a useful remedy for cats. Some types of fear in cats can be helped with Aspen – for instance when a cat is old, or ill, and the unconscious sense of his declining physical state makes him feel vulnerable. In this situation a cat can lose confidence and start to appear nervous although there's nothing directly frightening him. Aspen isn't a treatment for whatever illness may be affecting the cat, but can support his state of mind and help give strength to aid in recovery. Old cats can be helped to feel happier and more confident in their last phase of life.

CHESTNUT BUD*

Latin name: — Aesculus hippocastanum

Dr Bach's words: — 'For those who do not take full advantage of observation and experience, and who take a longer time than others to learn the lessons of daily life... they find themselves having to make the same error on different occasions when once would have been enough'

Keynotes: — **Immaturity, inability to learn from mistakes**

Goal of therapy: — **Increased focus and learning ability**

Chestnut Bud for People: Chestnut Bud is a remedy for those who find themselves making the same mistakes again and again, as though they never learned from their errors. In this state the mind is restless and impulsive, not fully engaged in the here and now. A person in need of this remedy tends to be easily distracted, absent minded, and often with a certain tendency to immaturity. Chestnut Bud is very often used for learning disabilities and problems faced by young people who find it hard to concentrate, often because of difficulty focusing on the present. This results in their being unable to retain information from lessons and life experience, so that they often appear to stumble from one situation to another without seeming to learn from life. People who need Chestnut bud are often driven by their emotions, failing to reason carefully and reflect on the effect of their actions and words. The remedy, taken over time, can help to reverse this tendency by allowing for better retention of lessons, whether taught in the classroom or in the 'school of life'.

Chestnut Bud for Cats: Chestnut Bud works for the cats in much the same way it does for people. This remedy is often useful in helping young animals that act quite impulsively and may be prone to making the same mistakes over and over. The remedy helps to increase focus and reduce the excessive spontaneity of their actions, encouraging more rational thought and concentration. Cats are capable of clear rational thinking, especially when this ability is well encouraged and stimulated. Animals in need of this remedy tend to be easily distracted, lacking in attention span and often forgetting the lessons of their training. Chestnut Bud has been observed to help these animals to listen more carefully and retain their lessons better.

Chestnut Bud is also a very useful remedy alongside Walnut, Elm, Larch, Cerato and Mimulus in helping young cats and kittens with their early learning and socialisation.

LARCH*

Latin name:	Larix decidua
Dr Bach's words:	'For those who do not consider themselves as good or capable as those around them, who expect failure, who feel that they will never be a success, and so do not venture or make a strong enough attempt to succeed'
Keynotes:	**Low self-confidence**
Goal of therapy:	**Emotional security and self-assurance**

Larch for People: Larch is for states of low self-confidence, a problem that affects most people at some time, and can cause a great deal of suffering. Poor confidence can stifle a person's whole life, sapping energy, spoiling relationships, stunting personal growth and delaying their trying anything new as they are convinced in advance that they would fail. A chronic lack of confidence may feel like a mild depression, where life holds no joy and the sufferer has no drive to do anything about it. In such instances Larch can be combined with other remedies such as Wild Rose, Wild Oat, and Mustard.

Larch for Cats: There are many circumstances where a cat can suffer from a lowered sense of self-confidence. Cats can lose confidence in old age, when they feel their strength, social status and ability to survive in the wild begin to slip away. At the other end of the age scale, a young cat can feel underconfident and insecure, especially if he hasn't been thoroughly socialised. A cat that is ill may fall into a nervous, anxious and insecure state of mind. Cats that are stressed by their environment, for instance by living with unhappy people or in a territory where too many cats are crowded together and vying for space, can also suffer a loss of confidence. So Larch can work in many situations, and together with many other Bach remedies depending on the circumstances.

HORNBEAM*

Latin name:	Carpinus betulus
Dr Bach's words:	'For those who feel that they have not sufficient strength, mentally or physically, to carry the burden of life placed upon them... who believe that some part, of mind or body, needs to be strengthened'
Keynotes:	**Mental fatigue and loss of concentration**
Goal of therapy:	**Restored mental energy and focus**

Hornbeam for People: This is a strengthening remedy for those times when the mind feels washed out, overtired and unable to concentrate any longer. The Hornbeam state often results from a period of hard work, especially mental work such as intense research or academic studies. People needing the remedy often feel unable to rise to their tasks any longer, badly in need of a mental and physical energy boost. The mind can become hazy and unfocused, listless and inefficient. The remedy helps to access reserves of mental energy, allowing greater focus and concentration.

Hornbeam for Cats: Hornbeam can be an important remedy to help cats through periods of stress or illness. In just the same way that it can help people, it can help cats to become more alive, alert and focused. It's one of the Bach remedies that can help maintain vital energy when a cat needs it most, for instance during convalescence or in fighting a serious illness. As Dr Bach wisely observed, the patients with the low mental energy or downcast spirits are the ones who often tend to cope less well.

If your cat suddenly starts acting very lethargically and seems mildly depressed, always check with the vet. Hornbeam can often help cats in a weak or vulnerable state, but it isn't a cure for the illness itself.

WILLOW

Latin name:	Salix vitellina
Dr Bach's words:	'For those who have suffered adversity or misfortune and find these difficult to accept without resentment… they feel that they have not deserved so great a trial, that it was unjust, and they become embittered'
Keynotes:	**Resentment and bitterness**
Goal of therapy:	**Ability to let go of negative feelings**

Willow for People: This remedy treats states of resentment, against other people, circumstances or life in general. This state can linger for years, and its sufferers can fall into a very depressed and despondent state. They can also become bitter and blame others for their unlucky lot in life. Often, the failure may lie with the person themselves and their feelings are quite unfounded. In other cases there may be a real reason for their sense of bitterness. Either way it's a very damaging negative emotional burden. The remedy helps the person to let go of this feeling, allowing them to put the past behind them and start afresh with a clearer mind.

Willow for Cats: In cats, Willow helps with a sense of resentment against specific others, or against humans in general, perhaps as a result of maltreatment. In the case of a cat that seems to dislike or resent people or a specific person, they may be frightening the cat without realising it, or else they may remind the cat of someone who was unkind in the past. This is often the case with rescue cats, who often may have gone through very unpleasant experiences. There are other Bach remedies we need to learn about to help with these kinds of cases, most notably Star of Bethlehem, an extremely important remedy that comes up later in the book.

Cats living together in a household can often develop disputes that may persist over time, just like chronic states of grudging resentment in people. These disputes are usually over territory, and the result may be two or more very stressed cats. The ill-feeling between them may not manifest itself in actual fighting; instead the war between them may be more of a 'cold war' of intolerance and mutual avoidance. In such situations Willow can help to iron out the resentment between the cats. Another remedy is Holly to help with jealousy.

BEECH*

Latin name:	Fagus sylvatica
Dr Bach's words:	'To have the ability to see the good within... to be more tolerant, more lenient, and understanding'
Keynotes:	**Intolerance and annoyance**
Goal of therapy:	**Opening up to tolerance and compassion**

Beech for People: The Beech remedy helps those who are overly critical and intolerant of others, always seeking to guide and shape other people's will. They have a very negative outlook, and to be in their presence is a very taxing, tiring, demanding experience. We all know people like this, who demand such high standards from everyone or seem to believe they're always right. It's a state of arrogance, constantly finding fault and highly judgmental.

The Beech state, though it's exasperating and annoying in another person, is actually a sad one, and there's often some underlying reason for its development. In many cases such a state comes on after a trauma such as shock, letdown or grief, if this hasn't been properly dealt with. The Beech attitude is also sometimes a means of self-defensive 'armouring', where the person mounts a shield between themselves and others. Beech lessens the tendency to criticise, and opens the mind up to tolerance and acceptance, to get in touch with hidden sadness and experiences that have not been released or dealt with.

Beech for Cats: Because the cat's mind is much less complex than ours, we only see the Beech state in a very simplified form.

Cats aren't arrogant or judgmental, negative or intolerant. However, one important use for Beech in cats is to help cats that have become untrusting of people as a result of unpleasant experiences. When all a cat has ever known of humans is fear, maltreatment, pain, loneliness and discomfort, he learns not to like or trust us. His unfriendly behaviour is simply a way of protecting himself from a type of animal (us) that experience has taught him is hostile and to be avoided. These kinds of traits are often seen in cats that have been abandoned or have run wild and end up in the cat 'rescue' system. Rescue organisations try to rehome the cats with caring families, but it sometimes takes more than love and care to teach the cat to adjust to life with people. Beech is one remedy that can help to soften their hardened attitude and help them learn to trust again.

CRAB APPLE*

Latin Name:	Malus pumila / Malus sylvestris
Dr Bach's words:	'This is the remedy of cleansing. For those who feel as if they had something not quite clean about themselves'
Keynotes:	**Personal shame or disgust**
Goal of therapy:	**Cleansing, acceptance, self-esteem**

Crab Apple for People: This remedy helps people who suffer from shameful feelings about themselves. They often feel a deep sense of uncleanliness, either relating to the way they look, the way they feel, or things that they have done – 'dirty', shameful actions. We are not talking strictly about guilt here – the emphasis tends to be on personal, often physical, shame, a strong dislike of some aspect of the person that they feel is nasty, unwholesome or ugly.

Crab Apple is also useful for humans feeling shocked or disgusted after dealing with nasty things. For instance, whether you are a veterinary nurse or a cat owner, looking after a very sick cat can be a hard experience, even if it's a cat you really love. You may be exposed to tasks, sights and smells that are not nice. Crab Apple can help to 'cleanse' these unpleasant impressions from your mind.

Crab Apple for Cats: Cats don't, as far as anyone knows, suffer from 'poor body image' or the feelings of shame, self-hatred and disgust that some unhappy humans do. Cats are lucky enough to be free of such painful neuroses. However, that doesn't mean we should disregard this remedy for feline use. Crab Apple has some useful physical applications with cats. Research has shown that combined with the other Bach remedies Cherry Plum and Impatiens, it can have a very good effect on skin problems. This effective combination is contained within the 'Rescue' Cream that is easily available from stores. This is the easiest and best way to use Crab Apple for such problems. It can help with allergic reactions such as 'hot spots' in cats, minor wounds and grazes that do not require the vet's attention, burns and stings. In itchy skin conditions where the cat is always scratching and damaging the skin, the cream can help to reduce the urge to scratch while promoting healing.

WALNUT*

Latin name:	Juglans regia
Dr Bach's words:	'The remedy gives constancy and protection from outside influences'
Keynotes:	**Impressionability from outside influences**
Goal of therapy:	**Protection and stability**

Walnut for People: Walnut is an important and frequently used remedy that helps with oversensitivity to outside impressions. This oversensitivity can manifest itself in a variety of ways: the Walnut 'type' may be over-susceptible to stress or upset in chaotic situations, and some people are easily prone to suffer from observing sad events or shocking news items on TV or unpleasant scenes in films. Walnut can help to reduce the intensity of their reactions to these influences.

Another manifestation of a negative Walnut state is where the person tends to be too easily swayed or influenced. This is similar to the Cerato state: they may be too easily taken by trends and fads, or too easily attracted to certain persons or movements. The remedy helps to promote the independence needed to detach oneself from these influences and gain a healthy distance from them.

Walnut for Cats: Walnut is an important remedy for cats. It can help in two basic ways. The first way Walnut helps is by offering strength during times of change. Cats are creatures that thrive on a consistent routine based around a stable territory. They don't like change, unless of course it's a nice new blanket to lie on or an especially tasty new kind of food! The changes that threaten cats are changes of territory or changes in the social group. When families move home, cats can be quite unsettled and many owners worry that they may not 'take' to the new environment. There are quite a few stories of cats making their way back to their former homes and resuming their old territory. Walnut can help them to readjust better to the new home and to assimilate the new environment so as not to go wandering off in search of more familiar ground. The remedy can also be useful in helping cats to accept a newcomer to the household, such as a new kitten or puppy.

Walnut is also important in situations where a cat's living environment is stressful, for instance living with a quarrelsome or unhappy family or in a crowded cattery where stress levels are high. This is extremely difficult for the cat. We mentioned earlier in the book that Agrimony can help here; Walnut is another useful Bach remedy in these cases. It's also highly important to reduce the levels of stress in the household or cattery wherever possible, to make for a more comfortable environment.

HOLLY*

Latin name: Ilex aquifolium

Dr Bach's words: 'For those who sometimes are attacked by thoughts of such kind as jealousy, envy, revenge and suspicion... for the different forms of vexation'

Keynotes: **Vexation, annoyance and jealousy**

Goal of therapy: **Compassion, tolerance and serenity**

Holly for People: Holly is another important and frequently-needed Bach remedy. Again, this remedy is concerned with how we cope with stress, and how life's experiences have shaped and moulded our personality. The person in need of Holly tends to overreact to any disturbance by becoming irascible and angry. Sometimes these overreactions are extremely powerful and violent, with outbursts of rage, physical aggressiveness, abuse, and impulsive or erratic behaviour. Less overt but just as psychologically destructive manifestations of this mental state are simmering hatred, jealousy and possessiveness.

Holly for Cats: Holly can also help cats with feelings of jealousy and vexation. These can be triggered by a variety of things. One example is when a new kitten is brought into the household and older cats feel resentful or threatened. This situation should always be carefully handled, but Holly can help the process of acceptance. Jealousy problems can sometimes emerge when owners have a new baby and suddenly stop paying attention to their cat – especially when the cat has had a very close rapport with the humans. There have been anecdotal reports of cats being found sitting or lying on a new baby's face, as though trying to smother it. Realistically, it's more likely that these cats have detected a source of warmth in the baby and that this behaviour has nothing to do with jealousy. The authors know of no verified instance where a cat has harmed a child out of jealousy – children do get scratched and bitten by cats, but usually because they have frightened him, pressed themselves on him or inadvertently hurt him.

Where this remedy can be of much use is in helping to reduce problems of aggression between cats. For a detailed account of this type of problem and approaches for tackling it, please see the section on Aggression in the next chapter.

STAR OF BETHLEHEM*

Latin name:	Ornithogalum umbellatum
Dr Bach's words:	'For those in great distress, great unhappiness, the shock of serious news, the loss of someone dear, the fright following an accident… those who for a time refuse to be consoled'
Keynotes:	**Sadness, shock, grief, past trauma**
Goal of therapy:	**Overcoming past hurts, moving on**

Star of Bethlehem for People: This is an extremely important Bach remedy that helps with sadness and despair, emotional trauma and shock. Star of Bethlehem is very effective in black, grim situations of loss and bereavement, the sudden death of a loved one or some other devastating impact that seems to tear our world apart.

Star of Bethlehem is also very effective as a retroactive therapy to help with trauma that lies back in the past, even as far back as childhood. As the release happens there may be dreams or emerging memories of the traumatic event. This is one of the more amazing properties of Star of Bethlehem, its ability to help people process emotional pain that has been buried for years and may even have been forgotten. In one case, a man in his 30s who had a phobia of water was cured with Star of Bethlehem. In dreams he remembered that as a small child he had nearly drowned. He couldn't remember this happening, so he asked his mother. She confirmed that he had had a very serious near-death accident in water at the age ofthree, which she had never wanted to remind him about as he seemed to have pushed it from his conscious mind. The Bach flower therapy was able to help with the upper 'layer' of the problem, his fears, but at a deeper level it removed from his unconscious mind the psychological scar that was causing the pain. There have been many, many such cases with this remarkable remedy. In another case, a woman who had suffered from depression ever since coming home to find her husband dead in the bath was cured after Star of Bethlehem was added to her therapy. She began to dream about the incident and was able to weep for the first time. As the daughter of a very strict soldier she had been brought up not to show emotions, and it was the buried emotional pain that was causing the depression. She was able to release the pain, and so the depression lifted. After seven years it had never returned. Star of Bethlehem is perhaps one of the most important remedies in Dr Bach's entire repertoire.

Star of Bethlehem for Cats: Star of Bethlehem works in very much the same way for cats as it does for people, and is one of the most important remedies in the entire Bach collection when it comes to feline care. One of its key uses is in feline rescue, to help with the rehabilitation and emotional healing of traumatised, psychologically scarred cats. The authors have often recommended that Star of Bethlehem should be given to any cat with an uncertain past, to help with any past problems that may have left a mark on the cat's present state of mind. Unfortunately, many cats suffer very bad treatment at the hands of humans, so 'past trauma' frequently involves maltreatment from past owners.

Traumatic incidents can befall even the best cared-for cat – attacks from other cats or from dogs, upsetting veterinary visits, accidents, and a thousand other unpleasant incidents. Whatever the cause, these are events that can all have a deep effect on the cat. Research has found that even if you give the remedies to treat the obvious emotional problem, such as a remedy for fear (e.g. Rock Rose or Mimulus), you often will not get full results until you also address the underlying traumatic incident. This is where Star of Bethlehem is extremely beneficial. Due to its uncanny ability to 'reach back in time' and address traumas that may have happened years before, it can help many cats whose problems all started after the unpleasant incident or period of their life happened to them.

WHITE CHESTNUT

Latin name:	Aesculus hippocastanum
Dr Bach's words:	'For those who cannot prevent thoughts, ideas, arguments which they do not desire from entering their minds... thoughts which worry and will remain and cause mental torture'
Keynotes:	**Lack of mental tranquility**
Goal of therapy:	**Restoration of inner peace**

White Chestnut for People: White Chestnut helps with a problem most of us have experienced in adulthood, if not as children. This is the feeling of having a seemingly endless train of unwanted thought spinning round inside one's head: maybe thoughts about bills or things that need mending, or things that are wrong with family relationships, problems at work, problems with the car, etc. Life is complex and full of niggling worries for most people, but for someone who needs White Chestnut it's even worse as they are unable to switch these thoughts off and relax. It can become a very tense state, resulting in insomnia and a damaging impact on daily life. The goal of the remedy is to help open up the mind to release that strenuous pressure. White Chestnut helps to dissolve this nagging feeling of worry, and restores inner peace to set the mind free.

White Chestnut for Cats: Mental tranquility is just as important for cats as it is for humans. Cats can suffer enormously from stressful states of mind, even if they don't (as far as we know) consciously work thoughts and ideas over in their mind. The remedy addresses the same underlying mental tension that affects our two species slightly differently. A cat that seems agitated, restless, unable to settle, constantly fidgeting or shifting about, may often benefit from this remedy's calming virtues. It's also important to check that no physical problem is affecting the cat.

RED CHESTNUT

Latin name:	Aesculus carnea
Dr Bach's words:	'For those who find it difficult not to be anxious for other people... they may suffer much, frequently anticipating that some unfortunate thing may happen to them'
Keynotes:	**Fear for others' welfare**
Goal of therapy:	**Emotional independence**

Red Chestnut for People: This remedy addresses a fear for the welfare of others. A person needing Red Chestnut has a tendency to worry excessively about their loved ones, often finding themselves imagining the worst things that could befall them. Often the nature of the state is that they are out of reach of that person, unable to help, powerless. This is the classic Red Chestnut fear: the other person is in need, and there is this rising fear that something horrible will happen to them. Parents with small children often experience this very unnerving feeling of apprehension, though it can also apply to many other situations. The goal of the remedy isn't to stop being a concerned parent, but rather to develop the ability to step back and have faith that everything will be all right. The message of this remedy is that life is too short to spend it worrying for no good reason!

Red Chestnut for Cats: Red Chestnut is an example of how the uses of Bach remedies for humans can mislead us to think too anthropomorphically if we aren't careful. For instance, one published book on Bach remedies for animals takes the remedy too literally by suggesting that it can make a mother cat less protective of her kittens. This is a misunderstanding of animal behaviour and how the remedies work. Any animal mother will naturally protect her young from a threat, such as a predator or someone who may want to harm the babies. Mother cats with young kittens naturally want to protect them, and will defend them with aggression if the situation warrants it. No amount of Red Chestnut will stop this natural behaviour!

However, this doesn't mean that Red Chestnut is never needed in feline care. The negative Red Chestnut state can arise in cats that have become too closely bonded to someone. This person is often their owner, who has allowed the cat to become too emotionally dependent on them – letting the cat be with them all the time, sleeping on the bed with them, curled up on their knee at every opportunity. This can cause a great deal of upset if the owner goes on holiday and the cat is forced to spend some time in the cattery. Even a five-star establishment won't compensate for the stress the cat may be feeling at the sudden disappearance of his beloved owner. Red Chestnut has a role to play in helping to reduce this anxiety; it would be advisable to give the remedy over a period of time and not wait until a week before the holidays begin!

PINE

Latin name:	Pinus sylvestris
Dr Bach's words:	'For those who blame themselves. Even when successful they think that they could have done better... they suffer much from the faults they attach to themselves'
Keynotes:	**Guilt and self-blame**
Goal of therapy:	**Acceptance and freedom from regret**

Pine for People: Pine is the Bach remedy that deals with one of the most painful and destructive emotions we know: guilt and regret. Guilt, or a sense of having failed or done wrong, places a terrible burden on the heart and heavy strain on our whole being. It can become impossible to find inner peace, and many sufferers become depressed and despondent.

People needing Pine may be feeling guilty for a real reason – there may be real deeds of wrongdoing they are responsible for, and they are troubled by the memory. In other cases blame may be taken on board by someone who is actually quite innocent, for instance if you blame yourself that an accident was your fault. Pine helps to let go of the past, while making amends. It allows a person to experience self-forgiveness, or to assess objectively whether or not they really can blame themselves for something. The ultimate goal, as always, is a lightness of the inner self and a good balance of the emotions.

Pine for Cats: The most important factor in examining Pine for cats is that, as far as we can tell, guilt or remorse are not a part of their emotional 'vocabulary' – this is one state of mind that they don't appear to share with us. Some owners insist that their cats have 'a guilty look' when they do something naughty, for instance when caught in the act of stealing some food from a plate. But a cat that freezes and looks unhappy when you catch him in the act doesn't look that way because he feels guilty. Instead, what the cat is probably thinking is that you are about to punish him, yell or shout – or, if people have mistreated the cat in the past, he may think you're going to kick or beat him. So this isn't a guilty state, but an anxious, fearful one.

So Pine is really more a 'people' remedy. Cat owners sometimes need it in those sad circumstances when cats are very old or sick, or badly injured, and have to be put to sleep by the vet. People go through a range of sad emotions when a pet dies, and one of the emotions can be guilt. People may feel they didn't do the right thing, or sometimes they start thinking about what they should have done to look after the cat better while he was alive. Most of these feelings are irrational, especially if you have been a caring and kind owner. But guilt hurts whether it's justified or not, and Pine can be an important remedy in these difficult times. By taking the remedy, people can come to an understanding that there was nothing they did wrong and nothing they could have done better; or, if they did do something wrong, for instance if some preventable accident was the cause of the cat's death, they can be helped to find self-forgiveness whilst making sure the mistake doesn't happen again.

HONEYSUCKLE*

Latin name:	Lonicera caprifolium
Dr Bach's words:	'Those who live in the past, perhaps a time of great happiness, or memories of a lost friend, or ambitions which have not come true. They do not expect further happiness such as they have had'
Keynotes:	**Longing for past happiness, nostalgia**
Goal of therapy:	**Letting go of the past, looking forward**

Honeysuckle for People: The Honeysuckle remedy helps people whose minds tend to dwell too much in the past. They are detached from the present, and also from the future, often believing that the best times of their lives are behind them and the present and future hold no possibility for happiness. Such people may want to show you old photographs or tell nostalgic stories from the past, always dwelling on events from long ago. There's often a kind of dreaminess to the Honeysuckle state, but where the dreamy Clematis state gazes out to the future thinking 'one day I'll be happy', Honeysuckle looks back thinking 'I was happy then'. The Honeysuckle remedy helps to ease this sad state of mind by helping to promote a sense of optimism for the present and the future.

One of Honeysuckle's major uses is in helping to heal the heartbreak after losing a loved one, where it works very well with other remedies such as Star of Bethlehem and Gorse. It's also a key remedy for helping the problems of the elderly, who often slip into a backward-looking state of mind where they are making no effort to enjoy life any longer. The goal of the remedy is to allow a person to continue holding on to past joys and happy memories, while at the same time opening up to the potential for life in the present and the future to bring more happiness.

Honeysuckle for Cats: Honeysuckle is quite an important remedy for cats. Just as it can help humans after a painful loss of a loved one, it can help cats that have lost their joy of life after losing a feline friend, or, as can also happen, a human companion. We have already learned that Gorse can help cats that have lost their spark of happiness after such a sad event. Honeysuckle is another remedy that can be used to help cats recover emotionally and move on.

Honeysuckle is also an important remedy to help with problems of separation stress that can occur when cats, used to constant human company, are left on their own for a period of time. This can be very distressing to the cat, even it's only for a short time. Honeysuckle, like the remedy Red Chestnut mentioned earlier, can help to prevent this problem occurring by encouraging the cat to become more emotionally independent.

WILD ROSE*

Latin name:	Rosa canina
Dr Bach's words:	'Those who become resigned to all that happens without any effort to improve things and find some joy... they have surrendered to the struggle of life without complaint'
Keynotes:	**Apathy, resignation, giving up the struggle**
Goal of therapy:	**Courage and determination to survive**

Wild Rose for People: Wild Rose is another important remedy, helping in situations of such unhappiness and emotional hardship that the sufferer feels paralysed, unable to rise above their problems any longer. It's a state of apathy, despondency and resignation to one's fate, all energy spent, resistance seeming futile. The person may start to withdraw into themselves, as though shying away from active involvement in life as the struggle hurts too much. To break out of this unhappy state they need to feel empowered again and to believe that they can do something to improve their lot in life. The Wild Rose remedy offers that spark of vitality needed to dissolve away feelings of apathy and enter a renewed phase of optimism and personal growth.

Wild Rose for Cats: Feline behaviourists talk about a type of cat behaviour called 'learned helplessness' which is very similar to the way people feel when they have become weary of struggling against life's challenges. Cats that have been exposed to chronic stress for too long can begin to 'shut down' emotionally: they may lose the will to survive, becoming passive and resigned to whatever happens. It's a frozen state where they have learned that they're quite helpless and there's no point in resisting. This state is often seen in cats that have been abused or treated cruelly for a long time. Cats that have fallen ill, or may be slowly dying, can also suffer from this state. Wild Rose is an important Bach remedy for such cats, as it helps to give them the strength to rekindle an interest in surviving and carrying on. One of its primary uses is in helping rescue cats, who may have often suffered the kind of hardships that have made them 'shut down' emotionally. It can also be very supportive to elderly, sick or convalescing cats. It works well together with remedies like Gorse, Oak, Olive and Gentian in helping to restore vitality to a depleted system. However, please remember that these are not medicines in their own right, and should not solely be relied upon if veterinary care is needed.

Veterinary associates of the Society for Animal Flower Essence Research have found that Wild Rose can be effective in helping injured wild animals, such as birds and rabbits, to survive the stresses of anaesthetic and operations. Very often these animals die on the operating table or soon after, not necessarily because of the injuries they've suffered but because the stress of being brought into a completely alien environment and handled by people is too much for them.This helps to give an idea of the potential of this remedy.

MUSTARD*

Latin name:	Sinapis arvensis
Dr Bach's words:	'Those who are liable to times of gloom, or even despair, as though a cold dark cloud overshadowed them and hid the light and the joy of life... under these conditions it's almost impossible to appear happy or cheerful'
Keynotes:	**Depression and gloom**
Goal of therapy:	**Optimism, light and joyfulness**

Mustard for People: Mustard's role is in helping with states of emotional gloom and dejection. A negative Mustard state can seem to descend like a black cloud, as though from nowhere, bringing a dark mood of depression that often can't be rationalised or explained. People sinking into this unhappy state of mind often lose all sense of joy and incentive, shrinking away from life and other people and lacking any mental energy to try to get back on their feet again. Mustard has been found to restore this incentive and help bring a little light back into their lives.

The Mustard state is quite closely related to the Wild Rose state, and the two remedies can work very well together if the person is suffering a feeling of apathy and resignation with no will to fight against their problems. It can also be very effective together with Olive, if the lack of mental energy and sense of prostration have come on due to energy depletion, for instance after a period of overwork or illness.

Mustard for Cats: Cats can also sometimes fall into states of depression, although whereas it often seems to happen for no apparent reason in humans, there's usually a clear reason for this emotional state in a cat. Causes can be too much stress, loss of a friend, change in circumstances such as being forced to leave a place that offers comfort and security, illness or a feeling of insecurity in old age. In any of these situations there can be a loss of joy in life and a reduction in motivation for the cat. Mustard, perhaps in conjunction with other indicated remedies depending on the situation – for instance Impatiens or Agrimony for stress, Walnut for unsettling changes, Honeysuckle for loss, Wild Rose for emotional 'shutdown' – can help to restore a happier state in the same way it can in humans.

If a cat has suddenly become depressed, isn't interested in food, and seems to be very listless, it's advisable to have his physical health checked by the vet. If the cat requires medical treatment, Mustard is just one Bach remedy that can be used to help him to recover; in fact as Dr Bach observed, helping the emotions may be a very important part of the cat's overall treatment.

SWEET CHESTNUT*

Latin name:	Castanea sativa
Dr Bach's words:	'For those moments which happen to some people when the anguish is so great as to seem to be unbearable… when the mind or body feels as if it had borne to the uttermost limit of its endurance, when it seems there is nothing but destruction and annihilation left to face'
Keynotes:	**Despair and faithlessness**
Goal of therapy:	**Hope and endurance**

Sweet Chestnut for People: Sweet Chestnut deals with a very dark, grim state of mind, perhaps the darkest that a person can experience. People in need of this remedy are plagued by terrible emotional suffering and morbid, bitter feelings from which they can't escape. This can happen during harrowing times such as the loss of a loved one, or in very painful and severe diseases where there is a dark and pressing fear of death. A Sweet Chestnut state can also be the result of an existential crisis, where the sufferer has driven themselves into a nihilistic depression by dwelling too much on the unanswerable questions of the human condition. For many, the idea that there is no meaning or purpose to life is too much to bear.

Sweet Chestnut helps to promote greater endurance, and a renewed sense of hope. Therapists often use it alongside Mustard for states of depression, and also in conjunction with Gorse and Star of Bethlehem. It can help to lighten states of extreme agony and help people get through the darkest experiences of their lives.

Sweet Chestnut for Cats: Luckily for cats, they don't have the capacity of humans to fall into states of existential crisis or depression associated with dark thoughts and ideas. They don't need to search for meaning in life, or understand 'what it's all about', the search for an elusive Truth that has tormented humanity for thousands of years. On a personal level this has created suffering and depression; on a global level it has given birth to religion, which in turn has created division, hatred and war. Cats are free from all this neurosis. They don't dwell on morbid ideas or begin to hate themselves. Their minds are much clearer, simpler, and in many ways healthier than ours. However, as sensitive and intelligent animals they are still capable of falling into very sad and anguished states of mind if they are sick, or left alone and abandoned, or suffering terrible neglect or stress. This is where Sweet Chestnut can be used to help them. A cat in need of this remedy may have experienced terrible hardships such as abandonment, cruelty or starvation. In other situations, cats may have lost a companion to whom they were strongly bonded, and be in a state of extreme anxiety over this. Cats that have suffered a great deal of physical hardship and are weakened as a result may need Sweet Chestnut and other remedies to help them recuperate and regain their strength and health. As in human therapy, remedies that may be chosen to work alongside Sweet Chestnut for cats include Star of Bethlehem (extremely important in helping rescued or previously maltreated cats), Gorse, Mustard, Wild Rose and Oak.

'RESCUE REMEDY' / 5-FLOWER FORMULA*

Keynotes: **All-round emergency and crisis formula**

Goal of therapy: **To relax, calm, soothe and support**

Dr Bach designed only one ready-made combination remedy during his career. It's a mixture of Cherry Plum, Rock Rose, Impatiens, Clematis, and Star of Bethlehem. This classic formula is probably the best known of all Dr Bach's remedies, and for many people it's their first contact with this system of therapy. Quite often, you may meet someone who has never heard of Dr Bach or his work, but who has often used this famous combination remedy and trusts its efficacy. Many people use this remedy for general nerves, if they have to take an exam, if they have to go to the dentist, have to travel by plane, if they have had an argument and need to soothe their nerves, or if they have had a hard day at work.

The simple idea of this combination remedy is to provide fast-acting relief in any acute, urgent, pressing situation. There may be no time to plan a treatment program or to choose remedies for the individual. The emergency combination is the 'first aid kit' of the Bach remedies, ready for instant use in a wide variety of scenarios.

Because there are various different companies producing versions of Dr Bach's remedies, there are a variety of replicas of the classic combination formula available. The original name 'Rescue

Remedy' is retained by Nelsons, while Ainsworths homeopathic pharmacy produces their version named 'Recovery Remedy'. While these are perfectly effective and able to deliver wonderful results, the authors favour the version produced by Healing Herbs Ltd, called 'Five-Flower Formula'.

Whatever version of the original formula is used, it's a very effective aid for a wide variety of problems suffered by cats. It can be used as a general anti-stress or calming remedy in all kinds of situations, and is a good thing to have around just in case of an accident or frightening event. If a cat is injured or suddenly falls sick and you are waiting for the vet to arrive or transporting the cat to the surgery, the remedy can be rubbed onto the gums or applied to the skin anywhere you can feel a pulse. The energy stored in the liquid will quickly find its way into the cat's system. For more information on methods of administering this and any other Bach remedy, see the chapter on *Practicalities of Giving Bach Remedies to Cats.* See also the section *Case Histories from the S.A.F.E.R. Archives,* which features a very striking case of a badly injured cat's treatment using the Rescue formula.

The various versions of the Rescue combination are also available in cream form, allowing some very interesting applications. Rescue or Five-Flower cream can be used as a safe all-round treatment for all kinds of skin problems, minor wounds, burns and aches. One of the most astounding cases the authors have come across with this cream wasn't a cat, but a pet bird that was flying around the owner's kitchen and accidentally landed in a pot of boiling soup that the owner was preparing for dinner! The bird's feet and legs were very badly scalded, with bleeding blisters and raw flesh. The vet didn't know what to do, and the bird was in such a bad condition that the devastated owner considered having him put to sleep to end his suffering. Everyone was concerned that, in any case, the bird would probably die of shock from the incident. As a desperate resort it was recommended that the owner tried applying some of the Healing Herbs 5-Flower Cream. Within *only one day* the healing of the bird's feet and legs had started, and after just a few days the bird was completely back to normal, showing no traces whatsoever of the incident. The vet is now quick to use the cream, as well as the liquid form of the remedy, in all kinds of cases!

There have been many, many cases of Rescue Remedy or 5-Flower Formula helping with emergency situations, acute fears, shock and trauma. However, because it's a generalised combination and isn't designed to take individual cases into account, you can create a much more flexible and individualised system of therapy by learning about the individual remedies and using them with skill and thought. While an effective combination remedy like this is a great thing to have in your pocket or at home 'just in case', the true satisfaction in using Bach remedies is to be able to choose from the whole range of remedies and become really familiar with the system.

Chapter Four

Bach Flower Remedies
in Specific Areas
of Feline Care

In this section we take a more detailed look into some specific types of problems and situations affecting cats and their owners, and the role of Bach flower remedies in helping them.

Aggression

Aggression between cats in the home is one of the more common feline behaviour problems. A certain amount of this may be play-aggression or mock fighting, an important part of a young cat's social education. Play aggression can also be directed at humans, such as when a cat will suddenly burst out of hiding and attack a passing ankle. Many have a favourite hiding place, and perhaps also a favourite victim! Such attacks are really carried out to sharpen and maintain the cat's hunting skills, muscle co-ordination, and control over each step of the stalk/pounce/kill sequence. Although most adult cats playing like this are unlikely to attack with full force, in some cases attacks can cause injury. By and large this is a normal behaviour that doesn't require any kind of remedy. Owners can be advised to carry a small toy, such as a mouse toy, with them to throw as they pass the cat's 'lair' to redirect his attention. What they *mustn't* do is try to deter such attacks by counter-attacks or use of force or violence, as pushing the cat away, etc., may be interpreted as reciprocal play and actually exacerbate the problem. The cat may also fight back rather than run away, which is obviously not a solution to the problem!

A more serious situation is where two cats compete aggressively over the territory they have been forced to share by being placed together artificially. For the same reason It can be very difficult (though not impossible) to introduce a cat into a home where there is already a cat in residence. There may be many fights, and the owners are often forced to rehome one of the cats. It's often a good idea to introduce cats when they are still quite young, preferably before they reach puberty. If a cat is already mature, it may accept a member of the opposite sex more readily. However, if the cats are neutered, the sex of the new arrival is often of less importance.

Treatment of aggression problems often involves castration or neutering, as when it occurs between two entire males. Some vets advocate the use of powerful psychotropic (mind-altering) drugs. The authors would urge readers never to consider the use of such drugs, as the potential side-effects can be very harmful.

Aggression is often the result of fear. Cats that are brought into a new home, or cats with a difficult past, e.g. rescue cats, may often feel the need to hide. This need should be respected. In normal cases the cat will gain confidence and soon venture out from his hiding-place, secure in the knowledge that it has a safe place to return to. However, chronically fearful cats may develop a secretive, absent lifestyle – perhaps rarely seen, only coming out when the coast is clear. Such a cat can become aggressive if attempts are made to force him out of his secure place. The aggression may be quite ferocious, as unlike predatory behaviour this will be not be play but rather an act of serious self-preservation. The harder one pushes the cat, the more aggressively he will defend himself, and injuries are likely to be quite severe. Confronting such a cat will also tend to lower the threshold of his aggression: he will tend to attack sooner, more ferociously and with less provocation each time. Certain Bach remedies can help with this kind of aggression, and also with the fearful state that underlies it. Treatment will have to involve adding remedies to food, which will be left out for the cat. Don't leave the food too far from the entrance to the cat's hiding place, and don't expect the cat to emerge until the coast is completely clear (children should be made to stay well away). In time, when the cat feels secure enough to do so, he will come out and investigate the food, thereby taking the remedies.

Bach flower remedies to help:

- **Beech:** To promote greater tolerance of other cats or people.
- **Cherry Plum:** To help reduce the strain of stress that may provoke aggressive behaviour.
- **Holly:** To help lessen the feelings of vexation and hostility.
- **Mimulus:** To help ease fear that may be the real cause of aggression.
- **Star of Bethlehem:** In case the aggression is partly caused by a past trauma or negative experiences.
- **Vine:** To help smooth out the urge to express dominance over other cats.
- **Water Violet:** Can help to promote greater social harmony amongst cats.
- **Willow:** To help calm states of resentment and hostility between cats in the home.

Bereavement

Like any other animal, cats are capable of states of grief and sadness when they lose the company of a friend or companion, either human or feline. Even though they are a less socially-orientated animal than a dog, cats can nonetheless invest a great deal emotionally into their companions and can feel very lost when suddenly left alone.

Bach flower remedies to help:

- **Gorse:** Can help to brighten the emotional state of a cat that is very downcast, broken-hearted or giving up the will to live.
- **Honeysuckle:** Can help a cat to recover emotionally from the loss of old friends and companions.
- **Star of Bethlehem:** To help cats recover from the shock of grief and loss.
- **Sweet Chestnut:** Similar to Gorse, to help bring some light into a very dark and bleak outlook.
- **Walnut:** Helps the cat to adapt to major changes in his life, giving strength and resilience to move on from the event and become happy again.

- **Wild Rose:** For cats that have fallen into a resigned state of apathy where they no longer care about anything.

Owners should also consider using Bach remedies at a time when a pet is very sick and has to be put to sleep by the vet, to help stay calm and composed during this difficult time. People bond closely with their cats and their passing creates a lot of emotional pain. Elderly people, who may have nobody else for company, can sometimes go into decline after losing a pet, and it isn't unknown for them to die soon after the pet. Bach remedies such as Star of Bethlehem, Gorse, Sweet Chestnut, Wild Rose and Mustard could help to prevent this from happening.

We also need to remain calm around a cat who is dying or soon to be put to sleep. Cats are very sensitive to our feelings and the emotional atmosphere, and if you allow the cat to sense that you are terribly upset and heartbroken, this could make his last few hours a time of stress and fear. If we can act calmly and peacefully, this will help the cat to leave this life in a more relaxed and reassured state of mind. This is a tribute of respect for the feelings of a loved animal that will soon no longer be with us. So for all these reasons it's important to use Bach remedies at a time of pet loss.

Car travel problems

Cats are not generally as fond of car travel as dogs, who often seem to adore it! However it's sometimes necessary to drive a cat somewhere by car – for instance to the vet, or to a cat show. Excursions like this can be very stressful to the cat, mainly because he is being taken off his territory to an unfamiliar place. The presence of the owner will tend not to reassure the cat as much as it would a dog. Cats can become habituated to car travel, and it's a good idea to introduce a young cat to the car early on in order to let him form positive associations with it. In addition to this habituation process, some Bach remedies can help with the stress of car travel for a cat.

Bach flower remedies to help:

- **Mimulus:** For general fears and anxieties; cats that whine and tremble in the car, and so on.

- **Rock Rose:** For cats whose fears borders more on terror, with panicky behaviour and perhaps scrabbling to get out. Cherry Plum could help here too.

- **Star of Bethlehem:** If fears and travelling problems have come about because of a past trauma associated with the car, e.g. an accident. This will help release the after-effects and the memory of the incident.

- **Rescue remedy:** As the three remedies above, Rock Rose, Cherry Plum and Star of Bethlehem, are all to be found within the classic combination formula, you could very easily use this instead for its effective calming effect.

Depression

Depression in cats is similar to depression in any other species, including humans. Symptoms may include vacancy and disinterest in life, loss of appetite, neglect of self-care and grooming, general listlessness and apathy. It should be obvious that any or all of these symptoms could be signs of disease, perhaps serious disease, and so a cat that appears 'depressed' should receive a medical check-up as soon as possible. As usual, once any possible medical causes have been dismissed, there is a potential role for Bach flower remedies. The remedies can also be used as a complementary treatment alongside medical care should this be necessary, to help support the cat and encourage recovery.

Unfortunately, conventional medical practice is rather quick to prescribe anti-depressant drugs for cats, mirroring the use of very similar drugs in human depression. While such drugs can certainly help to alleviate the symptoms of the imbalance, they are not curing the problem as they affect only the results and not the cause of the problem. At the same time, they are not a valid long-term therapy as they cause toxicity to the internal organs, particularly the liver and kidneys. Excessive use of such drugs is liable to create iatrogenic disease ('disease caused by the doctor'), often seen as skin disorders which are further suppressed with steroids, and so on, potentially triggering more serious and incurable states of disease.

It's important to ascertain what factors may have triggered the problem. Old age is a possible factor, where the cat is losing vitality. Another possibility is a traumatic experience, not necessarily recent. Yet another possibility is that depression has started after a long illness – the cat may have recovered physically but not emotionally.

An interesting fact worth noting is that indoor cats often eat spider plants. Although it is not poisonous, this popular decorative house plant contains a chemical that is known to have a euphoric effect when eaten. Cats deprived of grass (which free-ranging cats often chew) may nibble at the leaves, and will feel the effects of the chemical. Initially this acts as a stimulant, making the cat feel good; however, if the habit persists, the stimulating effects become less and less marked and the action of the plant can cause the cat to fall into a herb-induced state that closely resembles depression. To solve the problem, the cat's access to the plant must be prevented and steps should be taken to provide a more natural lifestyle for the cat. The cat may also benefit from homeopathic detoxification, such as a short course of Nux Vomica 6c (ask a homeopathic vet if in doubt).

Bach Remedies to help:

- **Star of Bethlehem, Wild Rose:** To help stimulate the will to carry on.

- **Gorse, Mustard, Sweet Chestnut:** To help uplift the cat's spirits.

- **Olive, Hornbeam, Oak and Gentian:** To help rekindle vital energy.

Emergency situations

Urgent or emergency situations in a cat's life may include many types of things, including:

- Being attacked by another cat;

- Suffering an accident;

- Experiencing a severe fright;

- Requiring urgent medical treatment and becoming highly stressed.

Each situation will have to be dealt with in its own way, but whatever the case Bach remedies can be used to help in two main ways:

1. To assist with the immediate problem and its psychological effect, for instance fear, terror, panic, distress, out of control behaviour.

2. To assist with the after-effects of the experience, helping to ensure that it doesn't remain lodged in the cat's psyche as a traumatic memory that could create all kinds of anxiety-related problems in the future.

Bach flower remedies to help:

- **Star of Bethlehem:** Star of Bethlehem is always the first Bach remedy we should think of when there has been any kind of traumatic situation, whether it's a recent happening or something that happened long ago. The remedy plays a crucial dual role in trauma management, having the unique ability not only to help an immediate problem but also to help prevent a recent traumatic incident from becoming a problem in the future. It's also a good idea for humans to take some Star of Bethlehem if they're involved in an accident or emergency situation involving their cat. The remedy is one of the key ingredients in:

- **Rescue Remedy/5 Flower Formula:** This classic combination remedy is intended for all emergency situations, such as deep shock following accident or injury, collapse, severe frights, etc. As well as the vitally important Star of Bethlehem this combination contains Rock Rose, Cherry Plum and Impatiens, all potentially capable in their different ways of significantly reducing the psychological distress of a traumatic or emergency incident.

- **Wild Rose, Gorse, Mustard, Gentian, Olive:** These would be used in the aftermath of the emergency, if the cat has lost interest in life and has become listless and apathetic. You should obviously have the cat regularly checked by the vet to ensure this is not a medical problem.

Fear and anxiety

Fear and anxiety are things we all know, and we can understand subjectively (without having to go into cat psychology) how deeply fear can affect our cats.

Fear comes in many different shapes and sizes. There are the frights that accompany traumatic events such as being attacked by another cat, or being in an accident. Long-term fearfulness may result from these incidents. Flower remedies can get to the root of the matter, helping to repair at an energy level the emotional damage that is causing the fear in the first place.

Bach flower remedies to help:

- **Mimulus:** This remedy addresses everyday, ongoing mild fears and anxieties. It isn't generally used for acute panic or very extreme fear or terror. People and animals that have developed mild phobias will often benefit from Mimulus. Larch could also be included here as it addresses lack of confidence.

- **Rock Rose:** Rock Rose is used for very extreme kinds of fear, terror or panic. It's quite easy to tell the level of fear in a cat. A very scared cat will either run as fast as his legs can carry him, stand his ground with displays of hissing, arching and ears laid flat, or may go into a frozen state of helplessness. In situations of very strongly pronounced fearfulness, Rock Rose is called for, perhaps along with Star of Bethlehem.

- **Five Flower Formula/Rescue Remedy:** This combination will be of great value in helping to calm acute states of fear, and is always worth carrying in your pocket 'just in case'.

- **Star of Bethlehem:** If you think that a fear or anxiety might have roots in a past traumatic incident or anything that the cat may have experienced before you knew it, Star of Bethlehem can be used to help with the emotional scars from the past that have not healed. Giving this remedy together with remedies for the present fear can be very effective.

Hyperactivity

This is very likely due to dietary matters or a lack of mental stimulation leading to boredom. Many types of 'hyperactive' behaviour can be a cat's way of expressing a stressed state of mind. A cat that has a healthy lifestyle, plenty of freedom and a secure territory will be far less likely to exhibit this kind of problem behaviour.

The following Bach remedies can help in some cases, but it's most important to isolate and rectify the real cause of this much-misunderstood problem. If the remedies don't help or only help a little, this simply means that you will need to look deeper to see what is causing the problem. It's always a good idea to check with the vet in case an overactive thyroid – one of the classic symptome of the disorder, is triggering feline hyperactivity.

Bach flower remedies to help:

- **Vervain:** May help for excessive exuberance and the tendency to use up too much energy.

- **Chestnut Bud:** For youthful impulsiveness, to help calm and mellow the cat's urge to run around like a mad thing.

- **Impatiens:** May help to calm nervous and highly strung animals that rush around. Impatiens can be very effective at helping to reduce stress and relax a cat.

- **Five Flower Formula/Rescue Remedy:** A general calming remedy

Kittenhood problems

Kittens and young cats can benefit from Bach remedies in a number of ways. Sometimes, remedies may be needed to help with problems that have arisen – these could include just about any of the problems Bach remedies are needed for generally, such as fears, trauma, or emergencies. Another important role for Bach remedies in helping cats at this delicate formative time of their lives is to help weld their personalities so they will be grow up to be psychologically strong, confident and well-rounded adults. Lessons learned and mental pathways developed at this early age will set the cat up for life, and so it's crucial to guide the process carefully and sensibly.

Bringing home a new kitten for the first time, we should be aware of how bewildered the little creature may be feeling. Unless born into your household, he will have just been parted from his mother and siblings, moved from the only place he's ever known to a strange and unfamiliar environment full of unknown creatures, sounds and smells. While some kittens seem to settle in without difficulty, others may be experiencing considerable emotional turmoil at this time. Make sure the kitten has plenty of rest in a secure place and isn't disturbed. Inquisitive and excited children should be firmly told to let him be until he settles. Children often exhaust a kitten by wanting to play with him all the time, so parents should keep their eyes open for this.

Socialisation is a vitally important part of the kitten's early formation. He needs to be gently introduced to a wide variety of experiences early on, in order to equip him with the mental 'software' to deal with any situation as he grows up. It's especially important to socialise the cat with people, adults and children, as well as other cats. See the section on Socialisation in the following pages.

This is a period of intense learning for the cat, and right from the start it's important to encourage him to learn positive lessons. The process needs to be shaped properly in order to ensure his development into a happy and well-rounded adult.

Bach remedies to help:

- **Mimulus and Larch:** These are important in helping to form a secure and confident personality in the kitten from the start. There's no harm in giving drops to the kitten even if he isn't necessarily showing signs of anxiety: reducing even the smallest feelings of nervousness will help at this stage to prevent future temperament problems.

- **Cerato:** Along with Larch, this remedy can help the kitten to form a strong, confident outlook. Together with sensible training – e.g. not allowing the kitten to become emotionally dependent on you – the remedy helps to foster a well-balanced and healthily independent spirit.

- **Walnut:** Sudden changes, such as being whisked away from everything he's known to find himself in an alien environment, can be unsettling. Walnut helps to strengthen the kitten's emotional resistance and allow him to adapt comfortably and confidently. Walnut also helps in socialisation, to help the young cat deal with all the new sights, sounds and places.

- **Elm:** This is an important remedy to help reduce the 'sensory overload' the kitten may experience when coming into his new home for the first time, and then later on during the crucial socialisation process.

- **Chestnut Bud:** Helps a developing mind to form positive associations and learn important lessons for life. The remedy fosters a young cat's intelligence, often appearing to sharpen cognitive skills and encourage quick logical thinking. An important early learning remedy.

Litter Tray Avoidance/Soiling in the Home

There are various reasons why a cat might fail to use his litter tray. It is important that the vet be consulted in order to eliminate any possible medical causes for the problem: the cat may be suffering from a digestive disorder, or a urinary infection. Once medical causes have been eliminated, it is safe to assume that the problem is a behavioural one.

Cats are very clean animals, and it is important that litter trays should be kept clean by removing stools and adding fresh litter regularly. Note that if the tray is kept too clean, emptying it completely each day and scrubbing it out, this can actually cause its own problems! The cat needs to be able to smell the scent of the tray, and it is this smell that will draw it back to use the tray again. If other areas in the home have been soiled and the cat has decided on his own toileting sites, eliminating the smell from these can encourage the cat to go back to using the litter. Areas can be cleaned with vinegar, and also with a strong alcohol such as vodka. Avoid using cleaning products containing ammonia, as these can actually attract cats (and dogs) to urinate in the cleaned areas. Another possible solution, once the soiled area has been cleaned up, is to start feeding the cat there – cats do not like to soil where they eat.

Cats may take to soiling in various areas of the house for reasons of frustration at not being allowed out, in which case measures need to be taken to provide greater stimulation. Owners should also be sure not to confuse simple urination with territorial spraying. Many cats live happily together, but sometimes there are frictions and some cats, especially entire toms, will redefine their territorial boundaries by spraying. Certain Bach remedies may help solve this issue (see below).

Stress of other kinds, e.g. nervousness, other cats coming in through a cat flap, etc., may also be involved. Sometimes, it happens that indoor cats are able to look out of the window and see strange cats coming onto their territory. Unable to get out and see the intruder off, they suffer from frustration and may begin to mark their territory inside, often by the window from which they saw the invading cat. The solution may involve a reconsideration of the cat's lifestyle, perhaps allowing it greater freedom. Simply covering up the window is not an ideal solution, but may be better than nothing as a first step.

The solution in general is to discover why the cat feels compelled to restate his claim on the territory. It may be necessary to have toms neutered (not a bad thing in itself, as there are too many unwanted cats already). Queens may also have to be neutered if they are attracting toms to the territory. Anxiety and frustration can be helped with Bach remedies, but we should remember that the cat is acting fairly normally and being put under rather unfair pressure. Rather than try to find a 'remedy' for this victim of human mismanagement, it may be better simply to try to offer the cat a more suitable lifestyle.

Bach remedies to help:

- **Impatiens, Agrimony and White Chestnut:** To help reduce stress generally.
- **Chestnut Bud and Rock Water:** To help encourage the cat to learn.

For spraying/territorial problems:

- **Holly, Willow, Beech and Water Violet:** To help smooth out the 'wrinkles' in the cats' relations and encourage greater harmony.

Obsessive-compulsive behaviours

Problems like self-mutilation, fur-pulling and excessive grooming often fall under the heading of Obsessive-Compulsive Disorders or OCDs. They are irrational, unnatural and compulsive behaviours apparently without a logical justification. In milder cases, cats may pull out large areas of fur, causing bald patches. Very often such behaviour is not an OCD at all, but caused by some allergic reaction, commonly to flea bites. More obvious OCDs are the distressing extreme cases where cats may chew at themselves and inflict injury. Self-mutilation of this kind is generally less common in cats than dogs. However, some cats appear to be very susceptible. Burmese cats in particular have been observed to claw at their teeth and gums until they bleed, inflicting damage to their faces and in some cases removing the skin from their face. Such types of behaviour are a serious problem and a sign that something is very amiss with an animal. Veterinary medicine has developed drugs to suppress self-mutilation behaviour, but as with all such drug therapies there are many pitfalls and drawbacks. Bach flower therapy offers a much gentler alternative; although owners are advised to seek medical help in OCD cases.

Bach remedies to help:

- **Impatiens:** Can help ease underlying stress and tension.

- **Cherry Plum:** Sometimes helpful in reducing the tortured state of mind that produces self-destructive behaviour.

- **Star of Bethlehem:** To assist in the healing of psychological trauma and scars that may have contributed to the development of an OCD.

If it transpires that a cat is pulling fur or licking excessively at skin due to a medical skin disorder such as an allergy, or the presence of parasites, certain Bach remedies may assist in solving the problem though they are not to be regarded as a treatment for the skin disorder itself.

- **Impatiens and Cherry Plum:** help to relieve the maddening itch.

- **Rescue/5-Flower Cream:** as a general salve to aid healing in conjunction with the vet's treatment.

Old age

Aging is a natural process that comes to us all, with the gradual and inevitable deterioration of the organism that has acted as host and vehicle to the vital spark that is 'us'. Just like humans, when cats reach a certain age they experience changes in both body and mind. Just when old age begins to show in a cat depends on two important factors:

- **General state of health:** a healthier cat will resist the symptoms of aging for longer.

- **Emotional stability:** likewise, a happy cat will tend go on for much longer before old age begins to take its toll.

Problems that commonly afflict the elderly cat include:

- **Fears and insecurity:** older cats often become fearful, anxious or confused. This can happen after a traumatic incident, such as an operation – which older cats may have to go through as their health weakens – or a frightening incident. As a result of anxiety, these 'old timers' may start to go downhill physically, with a loss of general tone and possibly a loss of resistance to illness.

- **Sense of vulnerability as physical power diminishes:** the weakening of physical powers can have an effect on the cat's mind, making this once strong and self-assured animal begin to feel underconfident and vulnerable. Sometimes, the onset of fears and anxiety is a sign of developing illness, so if an older cat displays an uncharacteristic loss of confidence, it's important to have him checked over by the vet, just in case.

- **Confusion and irritability as mental powers decline:** with the gradual loss of brain cells in the aging cat, thought processes can slow and behaviour can be affected.

Bach flower remedies to help:

- **Mimulus, Larch and Aspen:** To help with fears and loss of confidence associated with aging. Aspen may be especially helpful to help with anxiety caused by failing health, although it shouldn't be seen as a substitute for veterinary attention.

- **Star of Bethlehem:** Good to consider in case a frightening experience has been traumatic enough to affect the cat's confidence.

- **Oak, Gentian and Olive:** These remedies can all help to maintain the older cat's energy and zest for living. All three have a potential use to help the cat through periods of illness, when vital energy may dip.

- **Honeysuckle:** This remedy often helps older cats whose companions have died, resulting in a sense of loneliness and insecurity. (See the above section on Bereavement.)

- **Walnut:** Can help the older cat adapt to changes that come in the later stages of life, such as hierarchy shifts that result from his loss of power. Walnut may also help in adapting to reduced physical powers, such as the weakening of agility and stamina.

- **Mustard, Wild Rose and Gorse:** To offer support through times of dejection and reduced joy of life, and to help regenerate the will to go on.

Eventually, though, the cat is going to reach the end of the line. Bach remedies can do a great deal to promote a happy life for him while he is still able to enjoy it. However, sooner or later owners of elderly cats will have to face the decision whether or not it's in the cat's best interests to prolong his life. It would be cruel and pointless to try to depend on Bach remedies to keep a cat going if he is suffering. At that point we need to take responsibility to do the right thing if necessary. If we think it best to end the cat's suffering, we need to act quickly and decisively for his sake. Bach remedies can help us with that painful and difficult process.

Recuperation from illness

It's often forgotten that Dr Bach's main initial reason for developing the flower remedies was actually his interest in psychoneuroimmunology – the study of how the emotions affect physical health. Helping all living creatures to cope with illness is an important part of Bach flower therapy, even though the remedies are not themselves intended to cure diseases.

Bach remedies to help:
In fact, it's quite true to say that just about all 38 remedies can, in their separate ways, help to keep a cat healthy by generally promoting emotional happiness, confidence and vitality throughout his life. A happy cat will generally tend to be less prone to illness in the first place than a stressed or unhappy cat, and better equipped to deal with it if it should strike. However, if and when a cat falls ill for any reason, is injured or has to have an operation, there are certain key remedies that are often indicated to help him through this time and help promote healthy healing.

- **Gorse and Wild Rose:** To help against sinking spirits, despondency and loss of the will to go on.

- **Star of Bethlehem:** To help protect against the damaging traumatic impact of operations or other unpleasant experiences the cat may have to endure during illness.

- **Aspen:** To help the cat deal with unconscious fears and feelings of vulnerability associated with illness.

- **Impatiens:** To help the cat deal with stress and mental tension. Cats that have to be still and rested for a while, e.g. while a leg is in plaster or a wound is healing, can be helped to be more relaxed and patient.

- **Gentian, Hornbeam and Olive:** To help keep the vital energy maintained during illness, and help to promote a more positive recovery.

Rescue cats

It's a very sad fact that many cats are treated badly by people. The poor treatment these cats suffer from ranges from passive neglect to active cruelty. There are many ways that people are cruel to cats: by not feeding them, by making them suffer from terrible stress, and by physically harming them. Some very cruel people harm cats deliberately, for fun, sometimes killing them. Cats that survive these awful experiences are often very traumatised, afraid of people, or have turned aggressive. Some are completely undersocialised with people and even with other cats. Some have never been inside a human home and are understandably very wary of coming into the house.

Many countries have cat rescue organisations that deal with the victims of abuse and cruelty. They deal with:

- Cats that have been taken away from unsuitable owners by animal welfare organisations such as the RSPCA in Britain.

- Cats that have been abandoned because the people did not want to give them food or medical care, perhaps because they had simply lost interest in them.

- Cats whose owners could not cope with their behaviour or could not afford to keep them

- Cats whose owners have died and relatives rejected the animal.

- Cats that have run away from home and become strays or joined a feral group.

The work of these rescue centres and animal welfare organisations is to take the cats in, give them the appropriate care, and try if possible to rehome them with caring new owners in a suitable environment. This work can be very upsetting, as so many cats are emotionally traumatised or physically so damaged that there is little hope for them. They often have severe behaviour problems. These cats are called 'rescue' cats because they have literally been rescued from situations and environments that were adversely affecting their welfare.

Taking in a rescue cat is a challenge, similar to fostering a child from a difficult background, such as a war orphan. It is also an act of great kindness and goodwill, showing a deep love for animals. However, it's not for everyone. Ideally, someone who takes in a rescue cat should have good knowledge of cats – it may be unwise to have a rescue as your first cat. Giving the cat lots of care and love is important but even this on its own is often not enough to help a cat with emotional problems. Rescue cats, like rescue dogs, often turn out to be more of a handful than their adoptive owners had bargained for! The good news is that Bach flower remedies can often help with many of the problems of traumatised or abused cats. In fact this therapy is probably the best suited form of treatment ever developed to help with problems related to past trauma. By comparison, all the conventional medical world can offer are crude, often dangerous drugs that merely suppress the symptoms of the problem, often render the animal into a 'zombie' and may have all manner of unpredictable side effects.

Bach remedies to help:

- **Star of Bethlehem:** This is one of the most important remedies for all animals with a difficult past. One of the problems with rescue cats is that we often don't know what the cat has been through. Star of Bethlehem can be given to ANY rescue cat 'just in case' of past maltreatment and trauma. It's a very deep acting and fundamental remedy.

- **Mimulus and Rock Rose:** Most problems with rescue cats are due to fear. Experience of life often has taught them to be fearful of many things, especially humans. It's very important to use these fear remedies for such a cat. These remedies may have to be given to the cat for a long time, perhaps even forever in some cases. It may be that Mimulus or Rock Rose only partially help to reduce the fear of a rescue cat. This is often because they are only addressing the 'outer layer' of the problem, the fears themselves. If the fears are caused by a deeper problem, the past traumas experienced by the cat, Star of Bethlehem can be added to the cat's remedies to create a fuller effect.

- **Wild Rose, Gorse and Mustard:** These remedies can be needed for cats that have fallen into depressed states as a result of long-term traumatic life experience. Star of Bethlehem will also serve in this role, but multiple remedies over a period of time will tend to have a better effect.

- **Holly, Willow, Beech and Water Violet:** In all their various ways, these remedies can often help to soften the attitude of a cat who has only ever known humans as persecutors and tormentors. We may know we have the cat's best interests at heart, but the cat can only learn this slowly, over a period of time. It's up to us to show the cat that he can trust us. The role of the Bach remedies in this process is to gently work at the cat's emotions, allowing for that new trust to grow and develop.

Socialisation

This is a very important part of any cat's upbringing. Cats have to be socialised from an early age with adults, children, other cats and any other animals they may encounter, and with life's experiences in general. If a cat isn't properly socialised, he may grow up to be a fearful, difficult or edgy adult. Flower remedies can help with the process of socialisation, by easing some of the blocks such as lack of confidence, fears, and vulnerability to too many bewildering outside impressions.

Bach flower remedies to help:

- **Chestnut Bud:** To help the cat process new information and to learn from the experience.

- **Mimulus and Larch:** These two remedies would be very useful to give to any young cat being introduced to the world, people and other animals for the first time.

- **Elm:** This can help the young cat not to feel overwhelmed by the huge number of new sense impressions he's experiencing when you take him out into the world for the first time. For a cat that has never seen people, traffic, and all the busy world that we take for granted, it can be very emotionally tiring and even stressful. The remedy helps the cat to process all this new information without becoming too overloaded. This will also help a lot to create a confident and happy cat in the future.

- **Walnut:** This can help to 'shield' the cat from too many confusing impressions from the outside and help (like Elm) to let the cat process all the sights, sounds, and smells without stress.

- **Water Violet:** Can help the cat to bond to his new human carers, other members of the household and other animals that make up the new social group, whether these be other cats, dogs or other animals.

Chapter Five

The Last Goodbye:
When We Lose a Cat

One of the sad facts of having cats is that they don't live very long compared to humans. Even if all cats lived for twenty years or more, it would still mean that nearly every cat owner would experience the death of a much-loved feline companion at some stage. Every cat owner knows that the day will come when their beloved cat is no longer with them, yet when that day does arrive or approach, owners are often quite unprepared for it. Anxiety and hurt may be very considerable, to which are often added the additional responsibility of having to make the decision to end the life of a suffering cat.

In some countries such as Britain, there are helplines available for people needing emotional support after losing a cat or other pet. Helpline workers report that people can be so heartbroken at their animal companions' death that some of them feel suicidal. Many callers express to the counsellors that the animal's death has affected them more painfully than the death of a human friend or relative. Some people aren't comfortable about admitting this, breaking as it does our 'taboo' belief that human life has a greater value than animal life. However, if you feel this way it's nothing to be ashamed about: it just means that you loved your cat a great deal.

The role of Bach remedies in pet loss

Bach flower remedies offer a highly effective and flexible means of helping people to cope with sadness and grief at the death of a pet cat. Factors to deal with may include:

1. The shock of hearing of the pet's death, finding him dead or seeing him killed, e.g. in a road accident.

2. The impact of being told by a vet, perhaps completely unexpectedly, that the pet's life is coming to an end or that he's suffering greatly and it would be the right thing to put him to sleep. In both examples 1 and 2, a very helpful remedy is **Star of Bethlehem,** which helps to reduce the impact of the shock. Many people use the **5-Flower Formula** in such instances and find that it really helps them.

3. The guilt and regret associated with having to have an animal put to sleep, sometimes with self-blame at perhaps not having kept a closer check on the pet's health or safety. There may be mental torment over the sense of having neglected the pet's interests, perhaps at a time when other pressing issues to do with money/family/business etc. were presenting a distraction. Guilt and regret can also occur if the owner comes to believe that they may have acted too hastily, that something might have been done, that another vet might have been able to help, that the diagnosis/prognosis might have been incorrect, that they should have tried some other form of treatment, etc., etc. The negative effects of guilt and regret over past actions can be extremely damaging. The main Bach flower remedy to help with this is **Pine.**

4. Sometimes people have difficulties in making the painful decision to end things. Bach flower remedies, especially **Scleranthus** (and maybe **Cerato**) can often help with this kind of indecision, vacillation, swaying over this option or that. The person's feelings of guilt may also be a large part of the motivation behind such procrastination. There is also the fear that many people have of being deprived of the warmth of a pet's companionship or of being left alone. Unfortunately, if the cat is very sick and suffering a lot, the end result of hesitation is often more suffering for the animal.

5. The sense of separation and nostalgia after the death may be very prolonged and develop into severe depression in some cases. For these kinds of problems we have **Star of Bethlehem,** which is very important; **Gorse, Sweet Chestnut** and **Mustard** for feelings of despair and depression, and **Honeysuckle** for the feelings of painful nostalgia that prey on the mind. **Wild Rose**

can be important is people have sunk into a state of apathy and have lost the will to get up and get on with life.

The action of Bach flower remedies on grief

A frequently asked question is 'what's a good remedy for grief?' Let's examine this question, and what it means.

It should be understood that grief, as the outpouring of pent-up sadness, isn't only a natural process but also a very necessary one. Grief should not be suppressed, and to seek a remedy 'for' grief, that that will eradicate the symptoms of grief – just stamping them out so as not to have to face them – is wrong-minded. We shouldn't wish to 'blank out' the feelings we have for someone we have cared for. In one sense, the grief we feel is a way of paying tribute to the departed loved one, remembering how important their presence was to us. Through positive grieving we honour the legacy they have left us, the impression they have made on our own lives, and what we can learn from them.

Yet it does hurt, and we need to address the sense of devastation and pain. Bach remedies don't act as an emotional analgesic in the manner of a sedative drug; instead they are able to help with the process of expressing, integrating and then releasing pain. Once the pain is released, we can move on to enjoy the bittersweet memory of happy times gone by whilst also enjoying the present moment and looking ahead to the future. The remedies allow us to draw a balance between darkness and light: we mourn, but life goes on. A fine example of a healthy mourning process is the old tradition of the 'wake', especially as seen in Irish culture where the memory of the departed was toasted with much festivity and partying. This gives a good idea of how the different poles of sorrow and joy, light and darkness, can actually be healthily brought together in grief.

Releasing the pain in this way helps to prevent the first acute or 'inflammatory' stage of grief from dragging on too long, or from becoming deeply entrenched as a bleeding wound in the mind. People who have been so affected by the death of a pet or other loved one that they go on for months or even years unable to get over the sadness, need to work through the trapped pain that is torturing them, so they can put it behind them and move forward. Bach flower remedies are an important way to help this vital process.

Sue and Flo: a case of pet bereavement

Sue was told by her vet that her fifteen-year-old cat Flo, with whom she lived alone, had a tumour that was far advanced. There was not much hope for her; she was in pain already and the prognosis was poor. The vet had left the final decision to Sue, but there was little doubt that the correct course of action, for the sake of the cat, was to euthanise. Thus, Flo was put to sleep the same day, to spare her any further suffering.

At first Sue experienced a lack of emotional reaction, feeling quite numb and detached. For the first three days after losing Flo, she went about her duties as usual. After a week she began to feel a great sadness as though in a trance. Her emotions at this point were very stifled and repressed. As time progressed, however, a sense of increasing desolation came over her, which was most marked when she came home from work to an empty flat. In the months that followed, Sue went into a deep state of depression. Even her closest friends couldn't understand how she felt. It was as though a black cloud had settled over her and would not go away. She reported that she felt that her grief over Flo's loss was slowly crumbling away the edges of her life. It is notable that at no stage, pre-treatment, did Sue express her emotions through open grief.

A Bach flower therapist advised Sue to use the remedies Gorse, Wild Rose, Honeysuckle and Star of Bethlehem. Sue took these as directed, from a treatment bottle at 4 drops/4 times daily. Within two days of starting the remedies, she began to experience a sharper, more acute sorrow in place of the dull, numbing sense of pain she had been feeling in the aftermath of losing Flo. Suddenly she was releasing her pain through tears, and after two days of weeping she reported feeling 'amazingly light and refreshed'. Her dreams were very vivid, and in them she was with Flo again and Flo was well and happy, giving her a sense that she no longer had to worry and could get on with her life.

Sue had become very isolated in her depression, tending to avoid social company, and spending a great deal of time sleeping or randomly watching whatever happened to be on television. When she had been taking the flower remedies for about three weeks or so, she began to feel restless, as though she needed to get out and do things. There was the sense that she should not wallow in her pain, but rather learn from it and use the experience to reconstruct her life. A noticeable turning point occurred after the first treatment cycle (28 days) was complete, as Sue began to re-engage in social contact and positive activities. The depression having lifted, Sue felt she could move forward again. She now has two cats, with whom she shares her life very happily. Flo's picture hangs framed on her wall, and she touches it with a smile whenever she walks by. Now that the pain is fully released through the catharsis offered by Bach flower remedies, the emotions associated with Flo's memory have been transformed into something positive.

Chapter Six

Practicalities of giving Bach Remedies to Cats

Bach flower remedies are a very simple and easy form of therapy to use, and even the fussiest and most suspicious of cats can be given remedies without difficulty.

A word of caution

Before we go on, there's one very important rule to remember. In fact, the following is the one and only safety caution involved in Bach flower therapy for animals. As you will have seen, Bach remedies come in small bottles with glass pipettes from which the drops are dispensed. The first and most important rule of giving Bach flower remedies to cats (and other animals) and in fact the only safety caution in flower remedy therapy, is:

Never give drops direct from the dropper into a cat's mouth

This is simply due to the fact that the dropper tube is made of thin glass and could cause serious harm if bitten off and swallowed. Cats can move very fast, and may snap at the dropper if they think it's something to eat or if they feel threatened by it. The authors have never, in many years' experience, heard of a case of a cat or any other animal being harmed in this way, but it's nonetheless very important to follow this safety rule – just in case!

Methods of administering Bach remedies to cats

Bach remedies are usually (but not always) given by mouth. The easiest and most obvious way to do this is with a cat is by putting drops into a cat's food. How many drops should you give per day? Dr Bach described various methods of dosage, but the most normal dosage instructions with Bach remedies for people are to take about 4 drops, 4 times daily, either straight from the bottle or in a little water – so about 16 drops in all. The precise number of drops isn't vitally important, as long as the dosage is steady and consistent. As Dr Bach himself wrote:

> 'It *does not matter about being exact, as none of these remedies could do the least harm, even if taken in large quantities, but as a little is enough, to make up a small amount saves waste.'*
>
> (Collected Writings of Edward Bach)

Deciding how many drops to give a cat at a time depends on how often your cat eats. Most cats are given two meals a day, and so in such a case it's practical and effective to split the daily dose of 16 or so drops into two lots and give about 8 drops, twice daily with each meal. As with humans, there's no need to worry too much about dosage precision – the exact number of drops is less important than keeping up a good, steady and consistent dosage.

To give the drops this way, simply prepare the cat's dish with whatever food he eats – this should always be a good quality food that provides the cat with all the nourishment he needs – and then drop the drops on top of the food. They do not need to be absorbed.

Some cats may be in the habit of rushing in to start eating before you've finished putting the drops on the food. This should be avoided if possible, because of the potential risk of the glass dropper being bitten before you get a chance to withdraw it. If this is a problem, you could prepare the food on a kitchen worktop out of the cat's reach before placing the dish with added remedies on the floor for him.

If your cat only eats one meal a day, there is no problem with adding all the required remedies at once – remember that it's impossible to overdose.

Using treats

Outside of regular mealtimes, Bach remedies can be dropped onto little treats designed to tempt a cat, such as a small piece of roast chicken or a bit of raw meat if your cat will eat it. Remember, it's very unhealthy for a cat to be even slightly overweight. If you're feeding a cat a number of treats or snacks during the day as a means of getting the remedies into his system, cut down the size of his meals accordingly to make sure he isn't getting too much food.

Giving Bach remedies in drinking water

Cats as a rule drink much less water than dogs, but nonetheless they should always have a supply of fresh water available to them, especially if being fed a commercial dry cat food. This may present another way you can give flower remedies to a cat. It doesn't matter that the drops become more dilute by adding them to a bowl or dish of water. If Bach remedies were a traditional herbal remedy that works by the action of plant chemicals, diluting them this much would be a problem because it would weaken the concentration of chemicals and perhaps make them too weak to work. However, due to the way Bach remedies work, dilution isn't a problem. If desired, you can add 8 drops twice daily, or 4 drops 4 times daily, to a cat's drinking water.

Making a treatment bottle

Treatment bottles are a simple and practical way to:

1. Give several remedies at a time from the same bottle.

2. Save on remedies… and on cost!

3. Reduce alcohol content if desired.

4. Make remedies more palatable to cats by eliminating that unusual alcohol smell that cats may be suspicious of.

To make a treatment bottle, take an empty and clean dropper bottle (30ml is an ideal size, although 10ml will also do fine). Fill this bottle with fresh, clean water, preferably bottled mineral water (still, not sparkling). Add 2 or 3 drops of each remedy you want to use to the bottle, creating a tailor-made combination to suit the cat's requirements. Give it a little shake to mix up the contents and it's ready to use. Some people believe you should shake the bottle vigorously before each time you use it. Theoretically, this increases the 'potency' of the remedy very slightly, energising it by electrical friction; however it's not necessary to do this.

If you choose to add about 25% brandy or similar alcohol to preserve the water in the treatment bottle, at the normal dosage (of about 16 drops a day) a 30ml treatment bottle will last approximately 28 days. Alternatively, if you prefer to keep it alcohol-free, just keep the bottle stored in the fridge when not in use. The unpreserved water should last about 5 days, after which you can throw away any that's left over, and make another treatment bottle. Dosage from this treatment bottle is exactly as though you were using a 'normal' Bach remedy, about 4 drops 4 times or 8 drops twice daily. Again, don't worry about the extra stage of dilution, even when this diluted mixture is further diluted in water dishes. We are working with subtle energy here, not crude chemicals.

The wrong bottle!

A word of advice: don't forget to label treatment bottles, either with the name of the cat or with the names of the remedies! If you're giving Bach remedies to more than one cat in the household and you forget which treatment bottle is which, it'll be impossible to tell them apart. Alternatively, you could use bottles of different colour, e.g. a green one for Felix and an amber one for Tom... but it's probably easier just to obtain some of those cheap sticky office labels from your local stationer and scribble the cats' names on them. Do remember, though, that if you should give the wrong remedy to the wrong cat by mistake, no harm can possibly occur.

Sprays

Extending the idea of the treatment bottle, you can use the same trick to make a spray bottle. Bach spray bottles are a very handy alternative to giving remedies by mouth. These are useful when:

1. Cats are ill or unconscious and you're waiting for veterinary attention.
2. Cats are acting aggressively or hiding away in fear and can't be approached, e.g. rescue cats in catteries or rescue centres.
3. Cats are nervous in the car and it's not feasible to stop and give them drops in food or water.
4. Everyone in the household is a little stressed and could benefit from a remedy spray puffed into the air around them.

The mixture from a spray bottle will have exactly the same effect as usual. You simply pump a few puffs into the air around the cat, taking care not to alarm him. Tiny molecules of water containing the signature of the remedy will drift down; some land on the skin and are picked up by subtle electrical sensors, and others are inhaled into the system. When spraying, do not spray in the cat's eyes, nose or other sensitive areas. Spray lightly over the cat's head and around his body, at least a foot away. It makes no mess and can be done safely indoors.

Empty spray bottles can be obtained cheaply from homeopathic supply companies. To make one up, simply fill with still mineral water and add 4-5 drops of whatever remedy or remedies you wish to use. If the spray is to be kept for a while and used regularly, either keep it in the fridge or add 15-20% brandy to it to preserve the water. Some people like to add 1 or 2 drops of an essential (aromatherapy) oil such as Lavender. This gives the spray a pleasant smell and some oils also have a relaxing effect (a chemical effect unlike the effect of the Bach remedies). Note: do not put too many drops of essential oil in, as an excessive amount of some oils can cause headaches and other problems. ***Note: Adding essential oils also makes the spray mixture unsafe to use orally, as most essential oils are not suitable for internal use.***

Creams and lotions

The Bach mixture most often used on the skin in cream form is the classic combination of Impatiens, Cherry Plum, Star of Bethlehem, Clematis and Rock Rose, with the addition of Crab Apple. This enhanced 'rescue remedy' formula is available as Five-Flower Cream from Healing Herbs. It has many potential uses, including helping to heal burns and minor injuries, rashes and irritations, insect bites and inflammation. It has also been used to help cats with flea-bite dermatitis, an allergic reaction that many cats suffer from when they have been bitten by parasites. Five-Flower cream also contains almond oil and borax, which are known for their ability to help with skin problems.

You can also make a cream out of any combination of remedies you choose for any individual cat or particular problem. A few drops of one or more remedies can be mixed into jars of creams or lotions for rubbing onto the skin. A bland, neutral pH cream is needed for use on a cat's skin. Your home-made cream can then be used topically in just the same way.

The amazing acu-points

A surprisingly effective method of giving the remedies was first pioneered in Australia (by the Australasian Flower Essence Academy) and further developed for animal use by the Society for Animal Flower Essence Research. This fascinating method involves the use of a major cranial acu-point. This is an energy centre at the very top of the head, lying halfway between the ears of a cat (or cat, or horse). Energy centres around the body are the basis of therapies such as acupuncture, which are now scientifically tested and fast becoming part of mainstream medicine across the world. They are points where it seems we can connect with, or tap into, the many flows of subtle electrical bio-energy around the body.

Research has shown that topical application of flower remedy drops on this energy point on the head gives very effective results. Simply drop two or three drops of a remedy, or from a remedy combination in a treatment bottle, into the palm of your hand. Gently smooth the liquid into the fur on the top of the cat's head, taking care not to let any of it run into the eyes. This can be done very gently and discreetly during your regular 'cuddle' or stroking session. There's no need to rub the remedies into the skin, or for them to be absorbed. Ultra-sensitive receptor cells at the acu-point can detect the minute electrical signals from the remedy and 'read' the information. This method can be used several times each day just as one would do with oral doses.

The acu-point system has sometimes been known to be more effective than the more usual oral method of taking remedies. It also offers a brilliant advantage, in that it's perfect for giving drops to a cat that is sick, unconscious, or distressed. It avoids having to give the cat anything to eat or drink, which can be forbidden if the cat is due to have an operation in the next few hours. It's very simple and quick to wet your hand with a few drops and gently pat the cat's head.

Whichever method you use, keep giving doses of the remedies regularly each day. Consistency is the most important thing. Because the remedies are subtle by nature, they need to be given a chance to work. In most normal situations, it will take more than a day or two to see results and just giving a few drops one day and then nothing for two days will tend to produce poor results.

Giving remedies in an emergency situation

When giving remedies to a cat for acute shock, trauma, terror, or at a time of emergency, flower remedies can be given more frequently than the normal dosage. Drops may be given as necessary, perhaps every few minutes until the animal starts to calm down. Many people will use 5-Flower Formula as a general 'emergency remedy' in such situations. This is often very fast-acting and by keeping up a steady dosage of a few drops every few minutes it's often possible to calm a distressed animal.

If in doubt, or if you think the cat is injured or in pain, call the vet immediately. Cats that have become suddenly uncontrollable or aggressive for no apparent reason may have something wrong with them that requires urgent veterinary attention, and in these cases do not try to use flower remedies as a replacement for medical care.

If the cat is very frightened or in distress he may well not be interested in food or water at this moment. **Do not** try to put the drops straight into his mouth with the glass dropper. You could use a soft plastic syringe to get the drops in, or else simply rub some of the remedy by hand into the cat's gums and tongue, taking care not to get bitten if the cat is in distress. Alternatively use the acu-point method as described above, simply wetting the top of the cat's head with liberal quantities of the remedies until you can hand him over to the vet. Don't forget to keep taking drops yourself – if you can spare them – in order to keep a clear head during an emergency situation.

Chapter Seven

Frequently Asked Questions

In this chapter we'll recap on some of the points made in the book by setting out some of the most frequently-asked questions about Bach flower remedies and cats.

Question 1: How safe are Bach remedies to give to my cat?

If you've read the book, you already know the answer. However, let's remind ourselves again as it's such an important point: Bach remedies are very, very safe. They can be given to all cats, from the very young to the very elderly. They are safe to give to pregnant females or sick animals undergoing veterinary treatment. Not a single adverse reaction has ever been recorded with this type of remedy in over 70 years. They are hypoallergenic, drug and chemical free. It's theoretically impossible to cause any problems by 'overdosing' as the remedies are so safe and gentle in their action. If you give a remedy that isn't needed by the cat, the active constituents will simply fail to act. As Dr Bach himself said:

> 'As all the remedies are pure and harmless, there is no fear of giving too much or too often, though only the smallest quantities are necessary to act as a dose. Nor can any remedy do harm should it prove not to be the one actually needed for the case.'

> (Collected writings of Edward Bach)

Question 2: I want to give my cat Bach remedies, but he's on conventional medication. Is that OK?

This is an important question, as so many cats (like people) are receiving medication for one problem or another. Some herbal remedies can cause problems if given to a cat that is on medical drugs. These problems are called drug interactions, caused by the reaction of chemicals together. Such drug interactions can also be problem when one medical drug reacts with another, and with certain types of food. Doctors and vets (in theory, at least) are careful not to allow patients to suffer the negative effects of drug interactions.

But because Bach flower remedies don't contain chemicals or rely on chemicals for their therapeutic action, these drug interactions can't happen. This means that the remedies can't interfere with medical drugs. Bach flower remedies are also perfectly suited for use alongside other types of medicine, such as herbal or homeopathic medicine. Whatever else you use, or the vet prescribes for your cat, you can also use the Bach remedies freely. This is a very important and valuable property of flower remedies, which isn't found in many other effective natural therapies.

In many cases, using flower remedies alongside conventional medicine has not only proven to be safe, but has also helped the animal to need less of the conventional medicine by gently promoting a happier, healthier animal. This is especially true if cats and other animals have been suffering from physical problems as a result of stress, for instance skin problems that have come on due to emotional tension and are not too deeply established as chronic diseases in their own right. As long as the disease has not gained too strong a grip, and if the cat's immune system is reasonably healthy, helping to make the cat more relaxed mentally can gradually help to eliminate the disease.. This is such an important step for an unfortunate cat who not only has to suffer stress but also suffers the toxic damage of long-term medication with drugs such as steroids, which vets often give out much too easily with little knowledge of potential side effects.

Question 3: Why do the Bach remedies contain so much alcohol? Is that what makes them work, and is it toxic in any way?

The medium that carries the healing qualities of the Bach remedies is ordinary H_2O, plain water. Unfortunately, water doesn't remain fresh on its own, and unless preserved somehow it becomes a breeding ground for bacteria. Commercial Bach flower producers have mainly used alcohol – either grape alcohol or brandy, sometimes vodka – to preserve the water.

The alcohol content of the remedies in no way contributes to their effect. This can be demonstrated in different ways: firstly, the remedies still work when greatly diluted; secondly, they still work when given topically as opposed to orally; they work in sprays when they don't come into contact with the cat at all. Moreover, if the alcohol were having the effect, there would be nothing to differentiate one remedy from the other, and they would all work the same way. This is not the case.

Are there any health risks giving animals remedies containing alcohol? If we were giving cats any significant quantity of the remedies, the answer to this would probably be yes. However, due to the very tiny amounts involved if you adhere to the proper dosage routine, it's extremely unlikely that even over a period of years the alcohol content of the drops could have any significant toxic effect. There has never been any known case of this happening. If, however, you are concerned about the alcohol content of the remedies as they come straight from the bottle you purchase from your supplier, you can reduce the quantity of alcohol very significantly by making a treatment bottle as described in the previous chapter.

Question 4: How long do the remedies take to work?

In most cases of Bach flower therapy, assuming that the problem is a case for Bach remedies in the first place, and that the right remedies have been selected and properly administered, results are usually seen within two to three weeks, and sometimes much sooner than that. Naturally, results depend on the individual cat and the nature and severity of the problem for which he's being treated.

Interestingly, practice has shown that milder types of problems, such as everyday fears and anxiety, can take a little longer, perhaps two weeks or so, to be helped. Meanwhile, more severe and acute problems such as shock, strong fears and the severe anxiety of rescue cats with a history of being maltreated can often take much less time to react to the Bach remedies. Therapists and owners have often seen very frightened, nervous or fearfully aggressive cats become calmer within as few as 4 or 5 minutes. Remedies such as Star of Bethlehem and Rock Rose seem to be very important for gaining these fast and spectacular results. Remedies like Mimulus, which are for milder types of fear, generally do not work as fast. So, strangely enough, we can often predict that the highly traumatised rescue cat will show positive responses to the remedies sooner and more obviously than the relatively less stressed family pet. The same curious effect seems to apply to human Bach flower therapy: often, the worse the problem, the faster and better the effect of the remedies. A person suffering from terrible grief or despair can often respond sooner than a person with mild anxiety.

Question 5: How many remedies can I combine together at a time?

Only very occasionally will you need to use just one Bach remedy. In most situations, you will need to use two or more, and sometimes quite a few together. In fact, it's perfectly all right to use up to 6 or 8 remedies at a time.

As for what would be the maximum effective number of remedies to combine together, in truth nobody has ever really been able to establish this. One reason is that it wouldn't be ethical to deliberately give 20 remedies together to a traumatised cat to see whether they would still work. In such situations, you just get on with the business of helping the animal and leave scientific curiosity aside! In any case, it's not really important to establish a maximum number, whether it be 12, 15, 25 or 30 remedies, as it's normally (always, in our experience) possible to whittle the choice of remedies down to around 6 or 7.

Question 5: How long can I go on using the remedies? Are they OK for long-term use?

Because they're so safe, the Bach remedies are perfectly viable for long-term use if necessary. You can go on using Bach flower remedies for as long as required, and until you see their benefits firmly established and the problem as much helped as it can be. Because the remedies can't cause toxicity, it's impossible to overdose. Nor will pets become 'used' to their effect and require increasing doses to get the benefit, as can happen with drug-based treatments.

When people see their cats and other animals responding well to Bach remedies, their next question is often 'will I have to keep my cat on these remedies forever?' The answer is that, even if this should be necessary, it can't do any harm. In practice, however, it's usually not necessary to give the remedies for extended periods as they can have a very deep-acting curative effect.

For deeper problems, it may be wise to keep up the dosage of the remedies for a longer period of time, perhaps several months. Even when you see the problem helped, keep the remedies going for a while to make sure that the effect is well established.

Any necessary changes to the remedy formula/combination can be made at any time, allowing you to conduct an intelligent, well-structured and effective course of therapy.

Question 6: Can Bach flower remedies help with physical problems?

Yes and no. In his writings Dr Bach made the rather bold statement that all disease was caused by negative emotions, and that once these problems were helped, all disease would just vanish. It would be wonderful if it were true, but however, Dr Bach's idea should be taken with a large pinch of salt, as it isn't really borne out in practice. Unfortunately, this is the kind of sweeping claim that sceptical opponents of natural therapies tend to focus on to attack the credibility of the therapy generally!

So what is the truth – how far can Bach remedies help with physical illness? In lighter cases, when stress is causing minor physical problems that have appeared relatively recently and haven't become chronic, there's no doubt that Bach remedies can have a very good indirect effect on the physical level. For instance, many owners report that acute anxiety-related problems like colitis can be helped by using flower remedies. Research has shown that in many cases helping an animal on an emotional / psychological level to feel happier and less stressed can also have an indirect effect on physical health. We also know that Bach remedies have sometimes been reported to have a marked effect on certain physical problems, such as Scleranthus in helping with hormonal swings in females, when given for associated emotional problems.

However, in more serious cases of disease and in cases where the physical problem isn't stress-related, Bach flower remedies are really out of their jurisdiction and should not be considered the appropriate approach. Certain remedies like Gorse, Mustard, Olive or Wild Rose can be of complementary use in helping to boost an animal's vitality when ill. Animals that are very fearful due to their problem may also be helped. But the flower remedies will not provide the complete solution, by any means.

Even problems that were originally stress-related but have become chronic might not respond well to Bach remedies. For instance, ex-rescue cats that have suffered immune system weakness and chronic disease as a result of severe, prolonged stress in the past can benefit from Bach flower therapy for emotional and behavioural problems, but the remedies should not be relied on to treat their physical illnesses. We all want to use natural remedies as far as possible with our animals, and wish to avoid the use of conventional medicines for them as far as possible. However, if a pet is ill, home use of natural remedies should not be considered as an alternative to seeking veterinary help.

Question 7: I'm interested in using Bach remedies for my cat but I need to know that I can trust them. Do healthcare professionals such as vets and doctors recommend or use these remedies?

Yes, in many countries such professionals are using these types of remedies increasingly often, drawn to them for their simplicity of use, absolute safety record and high success rate. In Britain and the USA there are many veterinarians who favour Bach remedies as well as related therapies such as homeopathy. Associations such as the British Association of Homeopathic Veterinary Surgeons are growing all the time and promoting the use of these safe and effective approaches.

The Growth of Flower Remedy and other Complementary Therapy in the Mainstream – Some Facts:

- 30% of doctors in Denmark and Germany use flower remedies and other complementary therapies.

- As part of the growth of natural therapies in the mainstream, 20% of veterinary surgeries in the UK use herbal remedies.

- The Cuban Ministry of Public Health invited two Professors from Argentina to teach the first official course in flower remedy therapy to doctors and other medical professionals in 1997. By October 1998 there were 104 graduates, with 25 research studies showing notable results in treating various physical and psychological pathologies such as migraines, depression, skin conditions, menopausal symptoms, stress and asthma. Due to these encouraging results the Ministry of Public Health authorities officially recognised flower remedies in January 1999 as a valid medical modality to be integrated into the National Health System.

- Several scientific trials conducted by doctors in the USA and Central America have demonstrated significant reductions in depression on both the Beck and Hamilton Depression Inventories after flower remedy therapy.

- In Australia, flower remedy therapy is now being used in many major hospitals. One of its uses has been in special pain management units, helping with mental tension and resulting muscular tension and pain in patients recovering from major surgery who could not obtain full relief from opiate drugs.

- In Australia is it also now possible to take a University degree in flower remedy studies, and thanks to the pioneering work of the Australasian Flower Essence Academy (later renamed the LiFE Academy) flower remedies were successfully introduced into many Australian hospitals for use in special pain management centres.

- Adverse effects from the use of flower remedy therapy are unknown and have never emerged either in anecdotal reports or in scientific studies.

Chapter Eight

Bach Flower Remedy Combinations

The following are some suggested ideas for ready-made combinations, geared to suit specific situations and purposes. Following the instructions on how to make a treatment bottle, it's simple and straightforward to make up your own combinations (or 'combos') at home. By adding about 25% brandy or similar alcohol, it's then possible to keep the combos stored, ready for immediate use, for months. You can also add a new remedy to a combo at any time, allowing you to experiment to find the best recipe to suit an individual cat. As your expertise grows, you can very easily add to the list below, creating effective combinations of your own for any number of situations.

Post-Operation Combo

To help a cat to recuperate psychologically from an operation:

Clematis / Gentian / Impatiens / Oak / Olive / Rock Rose / Star of Bethlehem / Wild Rose

Show Combo

For those cat lovers who like to show their cats, and to help a cat that is stressed or nervous at a show:

Cherry Plum / Elm / Impatiens / Mimulus / Rock Rose / Star of Bethlehem / Walnut

Vitality Combo

A general aid to boosting energy and vitality:

Elm / Hornbeam / Mustard / Oak / Olive / Wild Rose

Rescue Cat

To help with a range of problems associated with past trauma or any negative experiences a cat may have suffered that are causing emotional problems in the present:

Beech / Mimulus / Mustard / Rock Rose / Star of Bethlehem / Wild Rose

Bereavement Combo

To help cats that are suffering from the loss of a companion or friend:

Gentian / Gorse / Honeysuckle / Mustard / Star of Bethlehem / Walnut / Wild Rose

Confidence Combo

A general aid to boosting a cat's sense of security:

Centaury / Cerato / Gentian / Larch / Mimulus / Star of Bethlehem

Travel Combo

For stress problems associated with car travel:

Cherry Plum / Elm / Impatiens / Rock Rose / Scleranthus / Star of Bethlehem / Walnut

New Kitten Combo (for the kitten)

To help a kitten settle into his new home and adapt to the unfamiliar environment as well as to aid socialisation:

Elm / Honeysuckle / Larch / Mimulus / Star of Bethlehem / Walnut / Water Violet

New Kitten Combo (for the other cat or cats in the household)

To help other cats in the household adapt more easily to any social upheaval caused by the arrival of the new family member:

Beech / Holly / Larch / Vine / Walnut / Water Violet / Willow

Group Harmony Combo

A general aid to creating a harmonious social environment for all the cats in the household. This could be given separately to each cat or used in a spray:

Beech / Cherry Plum / Holly / Water Violet / Willow

Veteran Combo

To help older cats with some of the common emotional problems they may suffer, such as loss of confidence and vitality:

Aspen / Gorse / Larch / Mimulus / Olive / Star of Bethlehem / Walnut / Wild Rose

Chapter Nine

Looking After Your Cat's Physical Health with Homeopathy

Bach flower remedies are a wonderful form of natural therapy but their use is mainly restricted to helping emotional/ psychological problems in cats, other animals and people. For cat owners interested in knowing about natural ways of helping their pets for a wider range of health issues, this section will briefly explore the uses of some homeopathic remedies in cat care.

What is Homeopathy?

Homeopathy has been developed over the last two centuries, based on the work of Dr Samuel Hahnemann (1755-1843), a German physician far ahead of his time. Homeopathy is a safe and effective form of medical treatment for a wide range of physical disorders (even the most serious ones, when skilfully used in the right hands). Homeopathic remedies are not drugs, cannot cause toxicity in the body, have no side effects as drugs have, and are fundamentally safe. With homeopathic medicine, you can rest assured that you can do no harm.

Homeopathy, like Bach flower remedies, is an energy therapy with a fast-growing body of hard scientific evidence to prove its effectiveness and great importance. In the face of the scientific evidence, some of which we outline below, it is no longer appropriate to be sceptical about the effectiveness of homeopathy. Professionals such as vets and doctors who continue to scoff at homeopathy, or refuse to accept it, or worse still 'don't believe in it', are either badly under-informed or unscientifically allowing their emotions to overcome their brains. As the homeopathic doctor Gabriele Herzberger writes:

> *'In scientific discussions, it is striking to note the extent of the ignorance of academics from the healthcare sector with regard to scientific studies on biological therapy. These professionals often fail to learn about the scientific basis of complementary therapies before developing critical opinions on the subject. Again, this violates the first rule of scientific enquiry, namely, the willingness to conduct unbiased investigation.'*

(The Fundamentals of Homotoxicology,
Gabriele Herzberger MD)

Giving homeopathic remedies to cats

Homeopathic remedies generally come in tablet form, in the shape of small pillules. There are various ways to administer them to cats. Unlike dogs, most cats will not readily take them from the owner's hand, and so the ideal solution is to add the remedies to food. Contrary to some popular myths about homeopathy, neither adding remedies to food nor handling them can reduce their effectiveness in any way. Like Bach remedies, if the correct remedy is chosen, it will help! The pillules can be crushed on a chopping board using the flat of a knife, and then the powdered remedy can easily be mixed into a dish of cat food. Alternatively, the softer types of pillules can often be dissolved in a little water to create a liquid dose that can be added to food. Some homeopathic pharmacies will provide remedies in liquid form on request.

Note: Some especially suspicious cats may be very wary of food that has been 'tampered with', and so it may be wise to add the crushed pillules or liquid remedies when the cat isn't looking! Once properly mixed in, the remedies should be undetectable and the unsuspecting cat will eat them up quite happily.

Potencies

Homeopathic remedies come in different levels of potency, ranging from low potencies such as 6c to higher ones such as 30c and 200c. The highest potencies are 1M and above, and these are probably best left for professional use as they are very powerful (even though they are actually more dilute!). The 'c' potencies are ideal for home use, with 6c and 30c being the most commonly available.

The general rule of thumb is that the higher the potency, the less frequent the dosage: so a 6c remedy could be given several times a day for up to several weeks, whereas a 30c remedy should be given less often – perhaps two or three times daily depending on the problem, and for a shorter time period. If in doubt, and for more serious problems, consult a homeopathic vet. In general it is always wise to have an animal checked by the vet even if you are intending to treat it yourself at home.

The following homeopathic remedies are easily available from homeopathic pharmacies and many health food stores:

Arthritis and Rheumatism

- ARNICA: The animal is in pain and does not want to be moved or touched. This is also a main remedy after an injury or accident.

- BRYONIA: Joints are swollen and hot, animal doesn't want to be moved or touched.

- CALC CARB: Weakness of extremities, swelling of joints (especially knee joints).

- CAUSTICUM: Stiffness and contraction of muscles. Good for older animals, whose gait is unsteady.

- CONIUM: Often helpful in the older animal, when hind legs give way.

- RHUS TOX: Stiffness, especially when weather is damp and cold. Animal improves on movement.

- RUTA GRAV: Joint pains that started after an injury. Like Rhus, the animal is better on movement.

(The first thing to think of with problems that may result from an old injury is ARNICA. One could give a combination of ARNICA/RUTA or ARNICA/RHUS depending on the case.)

Diarrhoea

- ACONITE: give at onset, especially if the animal has had a fright or a chill.

- ALOE: acute diarrhoea with jelly-like stools.

- ARSENICUM ALBUM: first choice in cases of mild poisoning (see the vet as well!). Can sometimes be helpful in cases of incontinence.

- CHINA: If diarrhoea persists and threatens dehydration. But the animal needs to be seen by a vet.

- LYCOPODIUM: used a lot in cases of chronic diarrhoea – a very good remedy for liver, acts chiefly on renal and digestive systems.

Gums and Teeth

This is a very important area of treatment. It's important to consider diet, as every animal needs a good diet in order to keep teeth and gums in order. It's also worth noting that symptoms such as bad breath/bad gums can be a sign of something more serious, such as kidney disease, so check with the vet to make sure that nothing serious underlies the problem.

- ARSENICUM ALBUM: A very good remedy for an animal that has actually been diagnosed with kidney disease and is suffering from oral problems such as gingivitis.

- CARBO VEGETALIS: Gingivitis that may stem from poor vitality, being run down, etc, often case with rescue animals.

- FRAGARIA: At 6x potency, twice daily, helps to get rid of tartar and plaque. The remedy softens the deposits to make it easier to scale the teeth. Use for up to 3-4 weeks before scaling or as a preventative measure.

- HEPAR SULPH: Abscess in the mouth, very painful to touch and bleeding easily. There may be a bad smelling discharge.

- KREOSOTUM: The mouth is infected and there is tooth decay.

- MERCURIUS: Sore gums, may be ulcerated, spongy, bleeding, receding.

- NUX VOMICA: Bad breath, possibly indicative of high internal toxicity. Most animals will benefit from Nux in any case, especially if they have been on a lot of conventional treatment. 6x or 6c potency recommended, with frequent dosage.

Kidney disease

This is common and serious problem for cats, especially older cats. The following remedies are often used successfully by homeopathic vets:

- ARSENICUM ALBUM: a very good remedy for kidney support, often indicated if the cat's breath is bad-smelling.

- EEL SERUM: one of the top remedies for kidney failure. Indicating symptoms include weight loss and a dull coat.

- PHOSPHORUS: useful in the early stages of renal failure.

Operations

- ARNICA: Can be given pre- and post-operation to aid healing and recuperation. Facilitates healing of bruises and tissue damage.

- LACHESIS: Experiments carried out by vet Dr Szumlakowski of Vienna show that Lachesis in 8x potency after operations is very beneficial. Lachesis raises physical strength, increases defence systems and helps prevent infection. Lachesis has a special effect on wound healing. Dr Szumlakowski has said 'nowadays I cannot imagine an operation without post treatment with Lachesis'.

- PHOSPHORUS: Useful if the animal may be (based on past experience, e.g. has been sick in the past) sensitive to the anaesthetic.

- RUTA GRAV: Together with Arnica, for any surgery on the teeth, as helps with repair of soft tissue. Also for healing after surgery on joints, repairs periosteum (covering of the bone), reduces the pain and speeds recuperation.

- STAPHYSAGRIA: Useful especially if the animal is to be spayed or castrated, have an amputation or organ removed.

Treatment procedure for operations

Many vets recommend Arnica/Ruta/Staphysagria 30c three times
on the day before the operation, and three of each again on the
day after the operation, adding three tablets of Lachesis 6x.
Consult your homeopathic vet before treatment.

Skin problems

Skin problems can be hard to treat because a chronic eruption on
the skin is likely to be a sign of some deeper problem. Causes could
be many: vaccinations, poor diet, stress, hormonal problems, or
allergies (which are in themselves a sign of a deeper disease).
Always start with a low potency for skin problems, as this is one
area where it is quite easy to cause an aggravation. The following
remedies are to help relieve some of the symptoms, though may
not entirely cure the disease causing them:

- ALLERGENS: Allergic reaction to inhaled or ingested allergens,
  e.g. airborne pollens, grass mowings, house dust, food. This
  remedy is not a cure, but may give some relief to the animal.

- ARSENICUM ALBUM: Skin hot and itchy, can crack or be flaky.
  The worst spot is often the back / tail area.

- GRAPHITES: The skin is very cracked, with a lot of scratching.
  Affected areas often skin folds behind joint, between pads,
  corners of the mouth.

- SEPIA: Alopecia from Ringworm. A very good remedy in
  treatment of all fungal and hormonal ailments.

- STAPHYSAGRIA: when a skin problem has come on after
  spaying, neutering or other operations, or when the original
  eruption was suppressed conventionally.

Thyroid disorders

Many cats develop overactive thyroid function (hyperthyroidism)
as they get older. A combination of the following remedies has
been found to be of frequent benefit to cats suffering from this
problem. Always check with the vet.

- FLOR DE PIEDRA

- IODUM

- THYROIDINUM

Urinary incontinence / Cystitis

(Here it's sometimes important to consider behavioural issues, because what is often classified as incontinence is actually a cat marking territory, or urinating out of fear/nervousness.)

- BERBERIS: Covers many kidney/bladder problems, such as kidney stones and cystitis. Often urine is bloody.

- BRYONIA: All ailments worse for movement; animal will leak urine while walking.

- CANTHARIS: A classic remedy for acute cystitis. Animal passes small drops of bloodstained urine with great frequency.

- CAUSTICUM: Important remedy for incontinence, especially in older animals.

- PULSATILLA: Often helps with females that become incontinent after spaying. Also animals that dribble urine when excited.

- STAPHYSAGRIA: Problems of incontinence after neutering (can be used preventatively around the time of the operation).

- THALASPI BURSA: Chronic cystitis. Symptoms similar to those of Cantharis, but not so acute (dripping less frequent).

Chapter Ten

Case Histories from The S.A.F.E.R. Archives

In this chapter we present some real-life cases to illustrate how Bach flower remedies have helped cats.

Case 1: The road accident victim

This case was reported to the authors by one of S.A.F.E.R.'s Veterinary Associates, Joanne Vyse-Killa VN:

A distraught owner rushed into the veterinary surgery one day with their badly injured cat. The unfortunate cat had been hit by a car and dragged some distance. Both of his hind legs were badly skinned; one had to be stitched along its whole length from ankle to stifle. However, the stitches kept bursting open, with the wound opening up to the extent that it was possible to see the exposed tendons. The wound refused to heal properly despite regular changes of dressing, and it was at this point that the vets, whom Joanne had long been trying to 'convert', decided as a last resort to try Bach Rescue Remedy. The combination formula was applied topically and regularly to the wounds. Within a week, the skin was growing back very positively; and after a second week, though still tender and healing, this distressing injury was almost completely better.

Case 2: A case of trauma

Elektra, a 14 year-old Siamese, suffered a traumatic attack by a neighbour's collie who had chased and cornered her. The dog shook the cat up considerably but inflicted no significant physical injuries (although he himself collected a couple of deep scratches to the nose!). The vet who examined Elektra shortly after the incident confirmed that she had been very lucky and was unhurt.

Though physically unharmed, Elektra soon showed signs of serious psychological trauma. Previously a confident cat, she became fearful especially at night. She appeared confused as to which exits to take to get from room to room or out to the garden, and, having been fastidiously clean prior to the attack, no longer seemed to know where her litter tray was or what it was for. She seemed to have completely lost her quality of life, and was depressed to the point that it looked to the owners as though she was 'waiting for death'. At the point where the owners contacted S.A.F.E.R., they were hovering on the brink of deciding to have her put to sleep as the kindest option.

Elektra was given a new chance by the Bach flower remedies. A S.A.F.E.R. practitioner discussed the therapy with her owners and together they selected a blend of remedies for her. These were Star of Bethlehem for the trauma, Wild Rose to help rekindle her vitality, Gorse for the severely depressed state she was in, Mimulus for her fearfulness, Clematis for the apparent confusion she was suffering from, and Larch for the loss of confidence. The remedies were prepared in a treatment bottle without alcohol and kept fresh in the fridge, the bottle washed out and renewed every five days or so. The drops were added to her food and additionally applied to the acu-point between the ears regularly each day.

After two weeks it was reported that Elektra was rapidly returning to her old self. Her confidence returned and the confusion and fears vanished. She came out of the depression so quickly that the owners observed 'it was as though someone had switched a light on'. The remedies were continued for a further two weeks, after which the therapy was stopped and kept on standby in case the symptoms should return. They never did.

Case 3: Night's unwanted companion

Night is a six-year-old black semi-feral cat whose owners, Jack and Helen, have had her since she was a small kitten. Night lives with them on a two-acre smallholding where she has always maintained a stable and uninterrupted territory. She is a very loyal cat, displaying almost dog-like characteristics in wanting to follow Jack and Helen and their dogs on long walks across the fields.

One day in early 2005, a black-and-white female feral cat started turning up, playing with Night and then disappearing again. Jack and Helen were pleased that Night seemed to have found a feline friend. They tried to befriend this new cat, but she wouldn't let them approach her.

Around Christmas-time, the black-and-white cat turned up again, but this time was keen for Jack and Helen's attention and would sit on the window-sill crying at them. She looked thin and not very well, and was clearly hungry. They began to feed her and she was treated homeopathically, after which her condition improved. At this point she moved in and they made a house for her in one of the barns. She was named 'Morse' for her peculiar squeaky, staccato call that sounded like Morse code!

Jack and Helen were happy that Night's friend was now part of the 'crew'. However, things did not go according to plan. Night suddenly decided that she didn't like the newcomer, and started refusing to eat. She wouldn't enter the building where Morse was housed, although it is forty feet long and has ample space for several cats. She was highly antagonistic towards Morse, and while previously she had been happy to play with her, now she would attack and spit viciously whenever Morse approached. Also very out of character, she would sit out in the rain all night and howl at the house. Worse still, within a few days she had started to show symptoms of a bad cold.

Night was given Holly for her resentment and hostility, Walnut for the sudden change in circumstances, and Water Violet to help promote unity, combined with some homeopathic remedies for her cold. These were all mixed together into a ball of lean minced steak – the only food she could be tempted her with in her peevish state!

Results were very quick. Within twenty-four hours the aggression was lessened, she began eating normally and would let Morse come a little closer without concern. Her cold cleared up remarkably quickly, the improvement in her mental/emotional state clearly contributing significantly to her overall recovery. At the last report, Night and Morse were playing happily together in the sunshine.

Case 4: Return of the King

Elvis was a seven-year-old tom who had once reigned proudly over his household but was now badly afflicted with a fear problem – whenever the doorbell rang, or if strangers came to the house, he would panic and run away and hide for hours. The problem had suddenly started about two years earlier, for no obvious reason. His health had been checked by the vet, who could find nothing wrong with him. The only thing the owners could think of was that, at the time the fears had started, there were builders in the house making extensive renovations. Since that time, the only place Elvis seemed to feel safe was his owners' bedroom.

Elvis was given the remedies Mimulus and Rock Rose for fears and panic, as well as Star of Bethlehem just in case something had frightened him during the time the builders were in the house.

A month later, Elvis was a different cat. He would come to greet visitors at the door and pay them a good deal of attention. People knocking on the door or ringing the bell would no longer send him into a panic, and he seemed perfectly at ease in any part of the house. His owner reported that 'it's as though he had been lost and has returned; now we have our dear old cat back again'.

This interesting case highlights once again the uses of Star of Bethlehem. Nobody ever knew whether Elvis' fears really were the result of the workmen's presence in the house. Perhaps one of them had frightened him; perhaps something had happened, e.g. a tool dropping on the floor near him or some other incident. It was impossible to know for sure. But the 'retroactive' quality of Star of Bethlehem makes it possible to address problems even if we don't know much about what happened, or whether it even happened at all. If we're wrong, and the remedy wasn't really needed, it will simply fail to act. If we're right and there was indeed a role for the remedy to play, it can reach into corners that no conventional treatment can even dream of.

Case 5: Past maltreatment

Harley was a very gentle, nervous and timid cat who needed a new home due to mistreatment by previous owners. His new owners, Gordon and Nickie, were interested in natural therapies and felt that the Bach flower remedies might help him to rebuild his life and learn to trust again.

As with many rescue cats, the details of Harley's traumatic past life were unclear. It was clear, though, that judging by his terrified reaction to men, he had almost certainly been severely maltreated by at least one man in the past. Harley had been seen by a vet and given a clean bill of physical health.

Harley had been with Gordon and Nickie for less than a week when they contacted a S.A.F.E.R. flower remedy consultant. When the practitioner arrived the cat was hiding under a bed and refusing to come out or eat. With the practitioner's guidance they gently sprayed a few puffs of Five-Flower formula under the bed and around the room, then left the cat in peace. When the practitioner returned the next day, Nickie reported that the remedy had had a very rapid effect on Harley. He had come out of hiding soon afterwards and ventured into the sitting room where he seemed much happier than usual sitting near Gordon and his brother, who was also staying in the house. The cat was also eating normally again.

At this stage, having seen such good results, it was decided that Harley could benefit from some more remedies to help get to the bottom of his troubles. He was given the following remedies in a treatment bottle:

- **Star of Bethlehem:** for the after-effects of unknown past experiences, to help him move on.

- **Rock Rose:** to help with his extreme fears and stress.

- **Larch:** to help restore his confidence and sense of security.

- **Beech:** to help Harley to redevelop a sense of trust in people.

- **White Chestnut:** to help ease the disquiet of a stressed mind.

One week later, the practitioner phoned to find out how Harley was doing. Nickie reported that only two days after starting the treatment bottle, the cat had walked right up to Gordon and jumped up on his lap to curl up and go to sleep. This behaviour was completely unheard of! Harley stayed on Bach remedies for a few more weeks and his whole attitude to people, especially men, softened dramatically. He was still slightly wary of male strangers, but not significantly more than any normal cat. In general, he was now happy and well adjusted.

Resources

Bach flower remedy suppliers

Healing Herbs Ltd
P.O Box 65, Hereford, HR2 0UW, UK
Tel: +44 (0)1873 890218
www.healing-herbs.co.uk
Healing Herbs Ltd produce the full range of Bach remedies as well as Five-Flower Cream. These remedies are made in strict accordance with the original method used by Dr Bach and are unsurpassed for their quality and the attention to detail that goes into their preparation.

Ainsworths Homeopathic Pharmacy
36 New Cavendish Street, London W1M 7LH
Tel: +44 (0) 207 935 5330
www.ainsworths.com
Ainsworths supply the full range of Bach remedies as well as a wide variety of homeopathic remedies.

Tortue Rouge Ltd.

Tortue Rouge produce a range of specially-designed combinations of Bach flower remedies for animals, helping with problems including separation anxiety, show nerves, past abuse, general fears and anxiety, and bereavement. The remedies, called Dr Petals' Elixirs, are 100% organic and have been found very effective in many cases.

Tel: +44 (0) 871 9008544

www.tortuerouge.co.uk

Readers in the USA can obtain the 38 Bach remedies from:

The Flower Essence Society (FES)
P.O. Box 459, Nevada City, CA 95959
Tel: 1-800-736-9222
www.flowersociety.org

Neals Yard Remedies
Neals Yard is based in the UK and distributes Bach flower remedies to many countries of the world.
Tel/Fax: +44 (0) 161 8317875
www.nealsyardremedies.com

Feline behaviour organisations

The UK Canine and Feline Behaviour Association (CFBA) is one of the leading feline behaviour practices and teaching centres in the world and is highly recommended to readers wishing to consult a pet behaviourist for any type of problem. CFBA advocate only the most effective and gentle methods and are vociferously opposed to the growing tendency for vets and certain feline behaviourists to recommend the use of powerful mind-altering drugs for animal behaviour problems.

CFBA also co-produce a range of excellent self-help videos, designed to empower cat owners to tackle many common behaviour problems in their cats, including separation anxiety, attention seeking and aggression. The films are written and presented by CFBA Chairman Colin Tennant, one of the world's top pet behaviour experts, and are available on VHS or DVD.

The Canine and Feline Behaviour Association
Tel: +44 (0)1442 842374
www.cfba.co.uk

Veterinary Associations

British Association of Homeopathic Veterinary Surgeons
Chinham House, Stanford-in-the-Vale, Nr. Faringdon
Oxfordshire, UK SN7 8NQ
Tel: +44 (0) 1367 710324
www.bahvs.com

American Holistic Veterinary Medical Association
2218 Old Emmorton Road
Bel Air, MD 21025
Tel: 1-410-569-0795

www.altvetmed.com

Education

The Animal Care College

Tel: +44 (0) 1344 628269

www.animalcarecollege.co.uk

Established for over 20 years, this specialist academy offers a wide variety of certificated and Open College Network-accredited home study courses in various aspects of animal care, including **Complementary Therapies for Pets**.

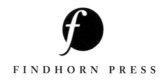

FINDHORN PRESS

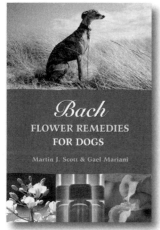

ISBN 978-1-84409-099-0

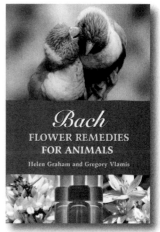

ISBN 978-1-899171-72-9

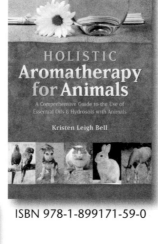

ISBN 978-1-899171-59-0

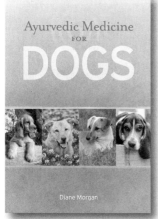

ISBN 978-1-84409-125-6

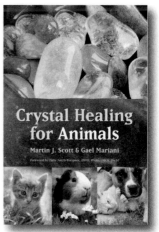

ISBN 978-1-899171-24-8

F I N D H O R N   P R E S S

Life Changing Books

For a complete catalogue,
please contact:

Findhorn Press Ltd
117–121 High Street
Forres IV36 1AB
Scotland, UK

t +44(0)1309 690582
f +44(0)131 777 2711
e info@findhornpress.com

or consult our catalogue online
(with secure order facility) on
www.findhornpress.com

For information on the Findhorn Foundation:
www.findhorn.org